Meta-Analysis for Psychologists

Richard Cooke

Meta-Analysis for Psychologists

palgrave
macmillan

Richard Cooke
School of Health, Education, Policing and Sciences
University of Staffordshire
Stoke-on-Trent, Warwickshire, UK

ISBN 978-3-031-73772-5 ISBN 978-3-031-73773-2 (eBook)
https://doi.org/10.1007/978-3-031-73773-2

Cover illustration: eStudio Calamar

This Palgrave Macmillan imprint is published by the registered company Springer Nature Switzerland AG.
The registered company address is: Gewerbestrasse 11, 6330 Cham, Switzerland

To Kayan, William & Alex

Preface

I started my PhD under the supervision of Dr Paschal Sheeran at the University of Sheffield in October 1999. Paschal had already authored several excellent meta-analyses estimating the magnitude of the relationship between intentions and condom use (Sheeran & Orbell, 1998; Sheeran et al., 1999) and during my time under his supervision he submitted his amazing conceptual review of the intention–behaviour relationship (Sheeran, 2002), which has been cited over 5000 times.

Paschal got all his PhD students conducting meta-analyses, such as Amanda Rivis' meta-analysis of descriptive norms (Rivis & Sheeran, 2003) and Tom Webb's meta-analysis of experimental manipulations of theory of planned behaviour constructs (Webb & Sheeran, 2006). Our research group also contained Sarah Milne, who authored a meta-analysis of Protection Motivation Theory with Sheena Orbell and Paschal (Milne et al., 2000), and Martin Hagger, who completed a meta-analysis of the common-sense model of illness (Hagger & Orbell, 2003) with Sheena. During my PhD, I was surrounded by researchers doing meta-analyses.

My first academic paper (Cooke & Sheeran, 2004) was a meta-analysis of correlations testing relationships from Ajzen's (1991) Theory of Planned Behaviour (e.g. attitude–intention, intention–behaviour relationships) done to test the question "Do properties of cognition moderate theory relationships?" We wanted to know if the magnitude (size) of correlations reported across studies varied depending on whether or not people scored low/high on properties of cognition like how stable variables were over time or how accessible they were in memory. This paper has now been cited more than 600 times—not bad for a first paper.

Twenty years since completing my PhD, meta-analysis has yet to gain mainstream acceptance within psychology. I think the main reasons for this hinge on two factors. First, until recently, you could not run meta-analysis in SPSS; I learned about meta-analysis by using Ralf Schwarzer's (1988) Meta programme before moving on to use bespoke software packages, like Comprehensive Meta-Analysis (Biostat, 2005) and metafor (Viechtbauer, 2010). Making psychologists learn about a new form of analysis using software other than SPSS has not helped meta-analysis become mainstream. Second, the lack of a textbook about meta-analysis written for a psychological audience; most of my training in meta-analysis came from either Paschal, Ralf's meta-analysis programme and manual, or discussing ideas with other psychologists who had run meta-analyses themselves. Learning about meta-analysis without a dedicated textbook has prevented meta-analysis from becoming mainstream in psychology.

Using the knowledge and expertise I've accumulated over the past 25 years, I aim to show you that meta-analysis is a technique that can be used to answer a research question **you're** interested in. The recent replication crises in psychology means publication of this book is timely as our discipline reckons with the need to test the replicability of results, something meta-analysis is well-suited to do. Meta-analysis is great at establishing the consistency or inconsistency of findings across studies and can help identify publication bias. I look forward to taking you on a journey of discovery that's probably quite different to what you've previously experienced.

Stoke-on-Trent, UK Richard Cooke
02 August 2024

Acknowledgments

I would like to thank Gina Halliwell, Emma Davies, Julie Bayley, Sarah Rose, Helen McEwan, Joel Crawford, and Andy Jones for their helpful feedback on draft chapters. I also want to thank Stefanie Williams for allowing me to reproduce a figure from one of her papers.

I would like to thank Palgrave Macmillan for their consistent support and patience throughout the production of this book. Particular thanks to Beth Farrow, Bhavya Rattan, Esther Rani, and Grace Jackson for seeing this book from inception to publication.

Finally, and most importantly, I want to thank Professor Paschal Sheeran for his guidance on how to conduct meta-analyses more than 25 years ago. I learned so much from Paschal in three years that has taken me almost 25 years to appreciate all he taught me. Without Paschal this book would not exist.

I have made every effort to trace copyright holders in the production of this book. If, however, any have been overlooked, the publishers will be willing to make the required arrangements to address this at the earliest opportunity.

Contents

List of Figures

List of Tables

1 Introduction to Meta-Analysis for Psychologists

Introduction to Meta-Analysis for Psychologists

Meta-analysis is the name for a set of statistical techniques used to pool (synthesise) results from a set of studies on the same topic. For example, in Cooke and Sheeran (2004), we extracted correlations reported by studies testing relationships from Ajzen's (1991) Theory of Planned Behaviour, for example, the correlation between attitudes and intentions and the correlation between intentions and behaviour. We used meta-analysis to pool results to provide a precise estimate of the magnitude (size) of these correlations. Such estimates can be used in many ways. We used them to test research questions in a later study (Cooke & Sheeran, 2013). Results from a meta-analysis can also be used to inform study design. Once you know the magnitude of a correlation you can use this information in combination with other information, including significance level and power, to determine the sample size needed for future studies. Pooled results can be compared to other pooled results to test theoretical questions too.

Who Is This Book For?

I believe meta-analysis can be made accessible to anyone who has completed an undergraduate degree in psychology. Meta-analysis builds on the principles taught about statistics used to summarise results from experimental and observational (survey) designs. Having completed an undergraduate degree in psychology, you already possess much of the statistical knowledge needed to learn about meta-analysis. The nuts and bolts of conducting a meta-analysis are similar to running statistical analyses you have already completed like t-tests, ANOVAs, correlations, regressions; you enter data into a dataset, label variables, and then ask a software package to analyse the data.

R. Cooke, *Meta-Analysis for Psychologists*,
https://doi.org/10.1007/978-3-031-73773-2_1

This book is also suitable for postgraduate students and researchers in other social science disciplines, such as criminology, economics, or geography who have had teaching on research methods and statistics as part of an undergraduate degree. Any discipline that uses survey data to correlates variables, or compares groups on an outcome, will be able to follow the examples in this book.

Why Is This Book Needed?

I believe that most postgraduate psychologists and many academic psychologists have not received training in conducting meta-analysis. This issue is compounded by existing books lacking examples that resonate with psychologists. In this book, I use examples from my published meta-analyses, and those of other psychologists, to show you how to run meta-analysis. I believe this book provides an accessible guide to meta-analysis that will help more psychologists to complete meta-analysis.

Aims of This Book

While systematic reviews are now an established methodology within psychology, meta-analysis remains under-utilised by psychologists. The main aim of this book is to demystify meta-analysis, making it more appealing to the average psychologist. Using the knowledge and expertise I've accumulated over 25 years, I aim to show you how meta-analysis can be used to answer a research question **you're** interested in. Another aim of the book is to showcase the benefits of running a meta-analysis. For instance, the recent replication crises in psychology means publication of this book is timely as our discipline reckons with the need to test the replicability of results, something meta-analysis is particularly well-suited to do.

Overview of the Book

The book is organised into four parts. Part I, 'Introduction to meta-analysis', introduces the basic ideas behind meta-analysis and comprises Chaps. 2 and 3. Chapter 2 outlines what meta-analysis is, what it involves, and why you should run a meta-analysis. Chapter 3 goes into more detail about effect sizes as understanding them is critical when conducting and interpreting meta-analyses. Part II, 'Preparing to conduct a meta-analysis', comprises Chaps. 4, 5, 6, and 7. Chapter 4 provides a brief overview of systematic review essentials around setting a research question, inclusion/exclusion criteria, and searching and screening. Chapter 5 covers data extraction for meta-analysis, with an emphasis on extracting effect sizes. Chapter 6 introduces quality appraisal for meta-analysis. Chapter 7 covers the idea of data synthesis, which is synonymous with meta-analysis. Part III, 'Conducting meta-analysis in jamovi', covers the steps you need to follow to conduct a meta-analysis in the open-source software jamovi and comprises Chaps. 8, 9, and 10. Chapter 8 introduces you to jamovi, outlining the steps you need to follow to be ready for meta-analysis. Chapter 9 provides an example of how to run a meta-analysis of correlations in jamovi and Chap. 10 provides an example of how to conduct a meta-analysis of effect size differences. Part IV, 'Further issues in meta-analysis', covers additional issues in meta-analysis. Chapter 11 compares fixed-effect versus random-effects in meta-analyses. Chapter 12 covers moderator (sub-group) analyses. Chapter 13 discusses publication bias. Chapter 14 covers extensions to meta-analysis. Finally, Chapter 15 provides tips on how to write up your meta-analysis.

References

Ajzen, I. (1991). The theory of planned behavior. *Organizational Behavior and Human Decision Processes, 50*, 179–211. https://doi.org/10.1016/0749-5978(91)90020-T

Cooke, R., & Sheeran, P. (2004). Moderation of cognition-intention and cognition-behaviour relations: A meta-analysis of properties of variables from the theory of planned behaviour. *The British Journal of Social Psychology, 43*(Pt 2), 159–186. https://doi.org/10.1348/0144666041501688

Cooke, R., & Sheeran, P. (2013). Properties of intention: Component structure and consequences for behavior, information processing, and resistance. *Journal of Applied Social Psychology, 43*(4), 749–760. https://doi.org/10.1111/jasp.12003

Part I

Introduction to Meta-Analysis

What Is a Meta-Analysis and Why Should I Run One?

2

What Is a Meta-Analysis?

Meta-analysis is the term for a collection of statistical techniques used to pool or synthesise results following a systematic review. Meta-analysis estimates the sample-weighted average effect size across all studies identified by the systematic review, providing a precise summary statistic that represents statistical information from a research literature. Meta-analysis also provides confidence intervals to show the range of possible values for the effect size, tests the statistical significance of the effect size (relative to the null hypothesis of there being no effect), estimates the heterogeneity of effect sizes across studies and assesses the extent of publication bias among included studies. The next section introduces several of my favourite meta-analyses to provide you with examples for further reading.

Meta-Analyses Conducted by Psychologists

The first meta-analysis I read was authored by my PhD supervisor, Paschal Sheeran, and Sheina Orbell (Sheeran & Orbell, 1998). This meta-analysis estimated the magnitude of the intention–behaviour relationship for condom use, that is, how big is the correlation between people's intentions to use a condom and their self-reported condom use across a set of studies? Using data from 28 samples identified following a systematic review, Paschal and Sheina conducted a meta-analysis that reported a sample-weighted average correlation of $r_+ = 0.44$. Following Cohen's (1992) guidelines for interpreting the magnitude of correlations (See Chap. 3) this correlation is interpreted as medium-sized.

What does this result tell us? It shows that across almost 30 samples, there is a significant, positive correlation between intentions and self-reported condom use; those who report intending to use a condom are more likely to report using a condom in the future than those who report they do not intend to use a condom. As

R. Cooke, *Meta-Analysis for Psychologists*,
https://doi.org/10.1007/978-3-031-73773-2_2

psychology studies are littered with correlations between variables and outcomes that are inconsistent, Paschal and Sheina's meta-analysis increases our confidence that intentions are a reliable correlate of later condom use. Such results are useful from both an applied and a theoretical perspective. Showing intentions consistently correlate with self-reported condom use gives interventionists seeking to increase condom use a target to modify in interventions. Results from meta-analysis also provide support for theorising, increasing confidence that intentions are a key predictor of behaviour as has been proposed for over 50 years (Ajzen & Fishbein, 1973) and continues to be proposed today (Michie et al., 2011).

The next meta-analysis I read was Chris Armitage and Mark Conner's (Armitage & Conner, 2001) meta-analysis of theory of planned behaviour studies. It is the dictionary definition of a highly cited paper, with more than 15,000 citations at the time of writing. The sheer scale of this meta-analysis still blows me away; Chris and Mark meta-analysed data from 185 studies—185! I've never meta-analysed more than 40 studies, and that took ages. It remains an impressive achievement and a useful resource for researchers looking for an overview of the theory of planned behaviour, although it is outdated now because many more studies have been published since this paper came out. Over time, meta-analyses need updating to ensure they reflect the results from a literature.

So good was Armitage and Conner's (2001) meta-analysis, I continued to cite it until the publication of Rosie McEachan and colleagues' (McEachan et al., 2011) meta-analysis. Rosie's meta-analysis focused on health behaviours, which meant that researchers could determine theory of planned behaviour relationships with reference to specific behaviours, like dietary behaviours, physical activity, smoking, et cetera. This is a key improvement over Chris and Mark's meta-analysis because they pooled results from across a range of different behaviours, which means their results provide a clearer picture of theory relationships rather than answering questions about the magnitude of relationships for specific behaviours.

As a health psychologist, it is helpful to know about specific relationships, for example, "How well do intentions predict drinking behaviour?" "How well do intentions predict dietary behaviours?" because it is these specific questions I am looking to answer in my own primary research studies. You must not assume that relationships are the same across behaviours. Indeed, Rosie's meta-analysis clearly highlights that intention–behaviour correlations vary between health behaviours (see Table 2 in her paper). This extra layer of specificity allows researchers to discern more clearly what the most important relationships are for different behaviours and estimate the effects they are likely to find in their own studies. A key goal of meta-analysis is to provide a precise estimate of effect sizes. A meta-analysis of studies for a single behaviour is necessarily more precise than one for multiple behaviours.

Rosie's meta-analysis remains the best health psychology meta-analysis I've read. It's a brilliant piece of work, providing behaviour-specific results that inspired my meta-analysis of theory of planned behaviour alcohol studies (Cooke et al., 2016). Rosie was only able to identify a small number of alcohol studies, so she pooled results for these studies with results for other substance use behaviours. I believe there are key differences in psychological drivers of drinking behaviour vs other substance-use behaviours. I used this idea as a rationale for my meta-analysis; I wanted to precisely determine the magnitude of theory of planned behaviour relationships regarding drinking behaviour, because that is one of my primary research interests. This is an example of where you can take an existing meta-analysis and create your own to answer a specific question. I'll continue to cite Rosie's paper until someone comes up with a better one, although like Chris and Mark's meta-analysis, it is also outdated.

Psychologists also run meta-analyses to evaluate the effects of experimental designs on an outcome, for instance, how well do experimental manipulations, like asking people to self-affirm before reading health information, affect information processing, intentions, and behaviour (Epton et al., 2015)? Such meta-analyses involve estimating the magnitude of the effect size difference (see Chap. 3) between two groups on an outcome.

For example, Peter Gollwitzer and Paschal Sheeran (2006) estimated the impact on goal achievement of forming implementation intentions (if-then plans), comparing results for those asked to form if-then plans with those not asked to form if-then plans in terms of whether they achieved their goal (or not), using an independent groups design. Following a systematic review, they pooled results from 94 studies and found an effect size difference of $d_+ = 0.65$ for forming implementation intentions on behaviour, a medium-sized effect size difference according to Cohen's (1992) guidelines (See Chap. 3). They have recently updated their meta-analysis, with results based on 642 (!!!) independent tests showing effect sizes for implementation intentions range from $d = 0.27$ to $d = 0.66$ (Sheeran et al., 2024).

Peter and Paschal also reported analyses based on behaviour type; they identified a sub-group of 23 studies that focused on changing health behaviour, with the effect size difference for these studies being $d_+ = 0.59$, which is also a medium-sized effect size difference. Both overall and health behaviour results show that asking individuals to form if-then plans is an effective strategy for goal achievement; these values are significantly different from zero, meaning that there is a significant effect size difference of forming versus not forming if-then plans across studies. Moreover, as medium effect sizes, effects are bigger than those reported for most psychologically informed interventions, which tend to be small-sized. Effect size differences provide useful information for those thinking about conducting studies; I can use the d value for health studies to estimate how many participants I need to recruit to find a similar effect size, when testing implementation intentions in a new study. Effect size differences and correlations are both examples of effect sizes, which we cover in detail in Chap. 3.

The final meta-analysis I want to cover in this section is by Stefanie Williams (nee Ashford), Jemma Edmunds, and David French (Ashford et al., 2010). They set out to test a precise theoretical question "How effective are interventions that target self-efficacy (i.e. one's confidence in performing a behaviour) for physical activity?" Self-efficacy is a key driver of behaviour in multiple models of health behaviour, most notably Bandura's (1977) Social Cognitive Theory. Stefanie and colleagues tested the idea that interventions led to increases in physical activity self-efficacy. They identified 37 samples and pooled results using meta-analysis, finding an overall effect size difference of $d_+ = 0.16$, a small-sized effect size difference using Cohen's (1992) guidelines. What was obvious from their meta-analysis was that results across samples for physical activity self-efficacy were heterogeneous, as can be seen in their forest plot (Fig. 2.1). Effect sizes were, frankly, all over the place: there were many small-sized effects, several medium-sized effects, some null effects, some negative effect sizes (i.e. where the control group increased their self-efficacy more than the intervention group) AND, one study with a large positive effect. Pooling effect sizes can show you results are less consistent than we'd like!

I've included this paper as an example of how an overall effect size from a meta-analysis is often the cue for more work on the part of the authors to understand what the results mean. In this case, Stefanie and her colleagues noted that heterogeneity between studies meant the overall effect size difference did not provide a helpful

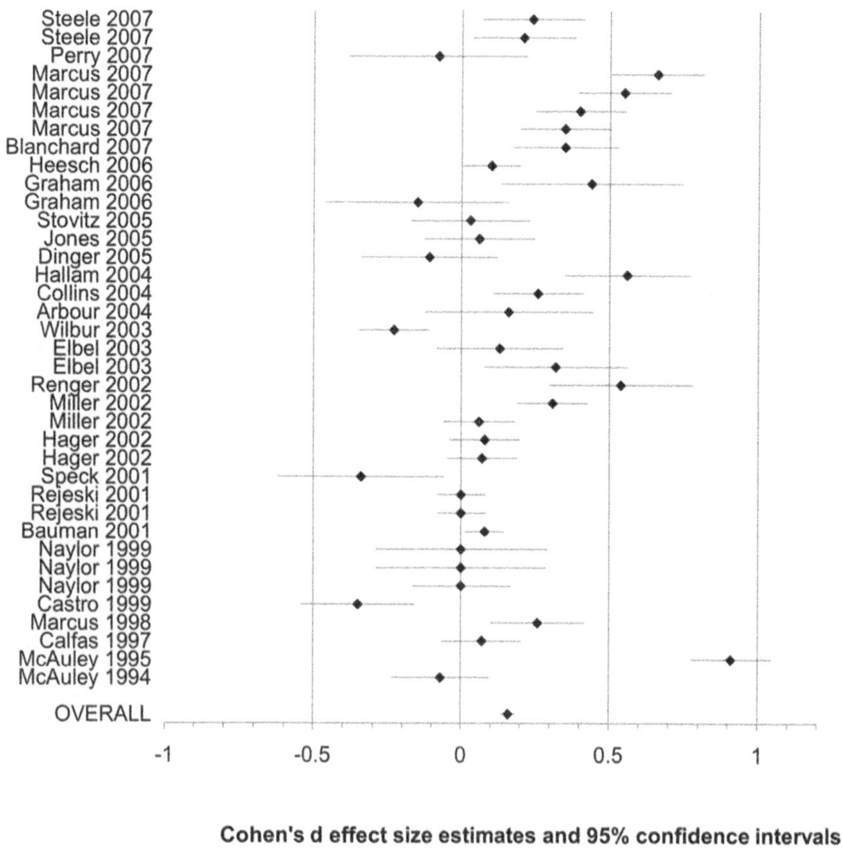

Fig. 2.1 Forest plot from Ashford et al. (2010)

summary of results. So, they conducted a series of moderator (sub-group) analyses, to account for the heterogeneity between studies.

One moderator analysis involved comparing results for studies that used/did not use different intervention techniques to increase self-efficacy; these moderator analyses allowed them to isolate the impact of specific intervention techniques to see if the technique was/was not, associated with changes in self-efficacy. The three techniques they tested were ones specified by Bandura as effective ways to increase self-efficacy: graded mastery (i.e. asking people to practise successful performance of the behaviour), persuasion (i.e. presenting information to persuade people they can become more confident) and vicarious experience (i.e. viewing someone else successfully perform the behaviour).

Stefanie, Jemma, and David found (1) studies that used graded mastery had less effect on self-efficacy compared with studies that did NOT use graded mastery and (2) that studies which used persuasion resulted in smaller changes in self-efficacy than studies that did NOT use persuasion. Both results go against theory and Bandura's suggestions and were surprising. Results for vicarious experience were even more surprising; studies that contained vicarious experience had a much larger effect on self-efficacy compared to studies that did NOT use vicarious experience.

The idea that vicarious experience was the most effective technique was apparently a mystery to researchers conducting the primary studies; vicarious experience was used in only nine of the 37 samples, with mastery used in 34 and persuasion in 33—the most effective approach was being used the least often! One of my favourite aspects of meta-analysis is its capacity to produce surprising findings that might be missed when evaluating the papers individually.

What Does Meta-Analysis Involve?

There are certain key concepts or ideas that you need to know to understand what happens in a meta-analysis. I'm going to introduce you to four concepts: (1) effect sizes; (2) pooling (synthesising); (3) sample-weighting; (4) publication bias. These concepts are important regardless of the type of meta-analysis you want to run and we'll return to them in greater detail later in the book.

What Is an Effect Size?

Effect sizes are the building blocks, currency, or units of meta-analyses. They are the result of a statistical analysis, like a correlation between variables, or an effect size difference testing the effectiveness of an intervention on an outcome or an experimental manipulation on a variable. Much of the time, meta-analyses are run using effect sizes reported by authors in a published paper. Sometimes, effect sizes are accessed from unpublished sources, including PhD theses, reports, or directly from the authors of the original studies. There are also occasions where the meta-analyst calculates the effect size themselves. In most psychological meta-analyses, the effect sizes are either correlations between psychological variables and outcomes, or effect size differences comparing an outcome between a control (comparison) group and an experimental/intervention group. I've already reported multiple effect sizes in this chapter including Sheeran and Orbell's sample-weighted average correlation of $r_+ = 0.44$ between intentions and condom use, and Ashford et al.'s effect size difference $d_+ = 0.16$ for interventions aiming to increase physical activity self-efficacy.

The choice of study designs you search for when you set out to conduct a meta-analysis means you will almost inevitably find studies containing effect sizes or the statistical information needed to calculate them—the only time this happens is when you cannot find any studies! So, a natural consequence of searching for studies that have correlated intentions with condom use is that such studies are highly likely to have reported the correlations you need for meta-analysis. Similarly, searching for studies using an experimental design or testing a behaviour change intervention means looking for studies that are likely to report the descriptive statistics, like means and standard deviations, you need to calculate effect size differences. So, if you set out to search for study designs associated with statistical information, that is, correlations are commonly reported in survey studies, descriptive statistics are commonly reported in experimental/intervention studies, you are well on your way to running a meta-analysis. Chapter 3 contains more information about effect sizes and Chaps. 4, 5, 6, and 7 cover all aspects of systematic searching, screening, data extraction, quality appraisal, and pooling results in meta-analysis.

What Does Pooling (Synthesising) Data Mean?

Pooling, also known as synthesising, means aggregating statistical information from multiple samples into a summary statistic, like a sample-weighted average correlation or sample-weighted average effect size difference. In meta-analysis, we pool results from different samples to produce a more precise estimate of the effect size; rather than rely on a single result or handful of findings from the published literature, we aim to pool results across as many studies as we can find as doing this increases our confidence in what the effect size actually is.

Meta-analysis pools effect sizes, like correlations or effect size differences, from a set of samples, treating each effect size in a similar way to how you average results from a sample of participants you collected data from to work out mean drinking intentions, mean IQ scores, or average screen time. Because meta-analysis is secondary study, that is, an analysis based on data that has already been collected, it takes the output of each sample, like the correlations calculated by the authors, and uses these correlations as the data points for an analysis. Hence, in a meta-analysis, each sample is equivalent to a participant in a primary study. So, you think about results in terms of how many samples you have, rather than how many participants you have, although you still report the total number of participants when writing up your results. Meta-analysts differentiate how many studies they included from how many participants were recruited into those studies by using different letters. You will be familiar with the idea of using N to report the total number of participants, and n to report a sub-sample, for example, how many young people we recruited in our total sample. In meta-analysis, we use K for the total number of samples, and k for sub-samples.

For example, in a meta-analysis, you might write: $K = 17$ studies were found that investigated the effects of behaviour change interventions seeking to promote health eating in primary age (4–11) school children. Studies were conducted in several countries, including England ($k = 4$), Scotland ($k = 3$), USA ($k = 3$), the Netherlands ($k = 3$), Norway ($k = 2$), and Slovakia ($k = 2$).

Pooling effect sizes achieves several important goals. Most obviously, it tells you the magnitude of the effect size across studies. Almost always, effect sizes vary between studies, and it is also typically the case that the pooled effect size falls between the highest and lowest effect sizes you find. Visualising all the effect sizes, typically by using a forest plot, that is, a graph showing the effect sizes from all samples with the pooled effect size at the bottom, helps us to spot outliers. That shiny finding, which is typically reported in a high impact factor journal, and often generates media buzz, will stand out like a sore thumb if all other samples find small or null effects. Running a meta-analysis will help you to avoid being too influenced by eye-catching results in particular samples, when evaluating your research literature. As we will see below when we talk about publication bias, it's very easy to be dazzled by a finding showing a huge effect of an intervention on an important outcome. Sadly, this bias pervades journals and psychologists are particularly prone to it (Chambers, 2017). Pooling results using meta-analysis is part of the solution to publication bias; if we pool results across studies, we can accurately assess the true pattern of findings from across the literature.

Pooling also increases the precision with which we can conduct future research studies. We can use the pooled effect size to estimate the sample size we need for future studies, leading to studies with greater power, that increase our confidence in results. We can use our pooled results to clarify to non-academic audiences what is going on and counter the sensationalism that sometimes surrounds research results.

What Does Sample-Weighting Mean?

When we pool results, we can either treat them as equally important or assign greater weight (influence) to some results and lesser weight (influence) to others. To treat all results as equally important is straightforward. Extract the correlations from studies you identify in a systematic review, then use any software package to average the correlations. As discussed by Borenstein and colleagues (Borenstein et al., 2009, 2021), such an approach has several disadvantages.

Meta-analysis is based on the idea of assigning greater weight to effect sizes with larger samples. This is called sample-weighting and is one of the key strengths of meta-analysis, helping you to see the wood from the trees. It's based on a straightforward idea from statistics; the larger your sample size, the more likely your effect size will generalize to the population effect size.

Here's a simple example. I often run studies to predict binge-drinking in English university students using psychological variables drawn from Ajzen's (1991) theory of planned behaviour. In these studies, I'm looking to correlate psychological variables with binge-drinking intentions. Imagine I have three research assistants helping me out with data collection. Each research assistant uses different methods to recruit students. Lee asks his mates to complete questionnaires and ends up with a sample of ten students. Debbie decides to advertise her study on social media and recruits a sample of 100 students. Ivy decides to ask her friends, advertise on social media, reach out to influencers, nag the chair of the university sports teams, and use every recruitment trick in the book to end up with a sample of 1000 students.

So, we have three samples that can be used to compute the correlation between drinking intentions and drinking behaviour.

Results look like this:

- Lee : $r = 0.80$ ($N = 10$)
- Debbie: $r = 0.65$ ($N = 100$)
- Ivy : $r = 0.50$ ($N = 1000$)

Which correlation should we view as most likely to generalise to the wider population of English university students? Based on the idea that the larger the sample the more representative it is of the population, we should trust Ivy's results more than Debbie's or Lee's, because Ivy's effect size ($r = 0.50$) is based on data from 1000 students.

Meta-analysis takes this principle to heart, which is why you end up with a sample-weighted average correlation rather than an average correlation. In practice, this means that each sample included in your meta-analysis is not treated equally; larger samples are given greater weight (influence) over the overall effect size relative to smaller samples. We'll return to this issue in later chapters, but a useful heuristic is that studies with larger samples sizes are assigned greater weight over the overall effect size calculated in a meta-analysis relative to studies with smaller sample sizes.

What Is Publication Bias?

Publication bias is the tendency of journals to preferentially publish papers reporting novel significant findings relative to papers reporting non-significant findings or papers that report replications of results previously published. Publication bias is endemic in academic journals and it's easy to see why; journal editors want academics to read their journal, in preference to reading competitor journals. One way to snag the attention of academics is to publish exciting, sexy, headline-grabbing results. Unfortunately, this approach is the antithesis of science, which seeks to uphold important notions like reliability and accuracy.

If journal's publication bias was restricted to editor's views, then I might accept it. But it is a malevolent force. Authors know which journals have the best reputation and seek to publish in these journals because they (rightly) assume that publishing there will improve their academic career prospects. This creates perverse incentives for authors. Imagine you conduct a high-quality study that shows no effect of your intervention on your primary outcome, kid's fruit and vegetable intake. Your intervention did, however, show an increase in another variable, like knowledge about fruit and vegetable guidelines. Now you know, due to publication bias, you'll struggle to get your well-conducted study into a top journal if you write up your null results for fruit and vegetable intake, so, maybe you are tempted to change the focus of the study and say that knowledge was all you were interested in. This is a wise strategy, if you want to get published in a top journal, but an awful example of science.

Null findings are just as important to read about as positive or negative ones. Knowing something does not change fruit and vegetable intake is a tremendously important result; it tells readers that this intervention might not be the golden ticket to success and should cause them (and the authors!) to reflect on why the intervention did not change the primary outcome. Let's face it, changing behaviour is hard, and I truly believe it is easier to change other things like knowledge, beliefs, scores on a test, so let's not make a song and dance when we achieve something that is (relatively) easy. Publication bias will always exist, in my opinion. The incentives to present results in a way that favours publication are not going away, and publication in a top journal is an activity that produces major benefits for authors. While I fully support Open Science initiatives, like pre-registering studies, I believe there will always be those who seek to game the system.

Why does publication bias matter in a meta-analysis? Well, when you conduct a meta-analysis, you are looking to pool results from across the literature: positive, negative, and null. Because meta-analysts know about publication bias, they expect that pooled results are likely to over-represent positive findings, as these findings are more likely to find their way into the published literature you search. Meta-analysts have created two countermeasures to publication bias, statistics estimating the extent of publication bias and funnel plots. When you conduct a meta-analysis, your output contains estimates of publication bias and funnel plots to allow you to interpret the extent of publication bias in your included samples. We'll go into more detail on publication bias later in the book (see Chap. 13).

Why Should I Run a Meta-Analysis?

I think there are several reasons to run a meta-analysis:

- To provide precise estimate(s) of effect size(s)
- To address theoretical or applied research questions

- To generate research hypotheses/questions for future studies

Meta-analysis' primary aim is to provide a precise estimate of an effect size across a literature. Beyond the immediate goal of being something to report in an academic paper, this precise estimate can serve as a guide to future primary research. For example, when designing a study, researchers often want to know how many participants to recruit. One of the three pieces of statistical information you need to accurately calculate a sample size is the effect size you expect to find. So, you can use the effect size reported from a meta-analysis of studies like the study you want to conduct to base your sample size calculation on. The effect size is often the hardest part to determine of the sample size calculation as most researchers typically set their significance (alpha) and power to default levels ($p < 0.05$ for alpha and 0.8 for power). I have used Gollwitzer and Sheeran's (2006) effect size difference of $d_+ = 0.59$ for health studies using implementation intentions as part of sample size calculations. I feel more confident doing this than the alternative, which is to sample (cherry pick) a few studies that are like what we want to do and use those as a guide, often (magically) finding that the smallest sample size from a similar study is the one we'll use!

In many disciplines, the precision afforded by meta-analysis is taken extremely seriously. If you type 'evidence pyramid' into a search engine you will see a hierarchy of study designs used in epidemiology, medicine, and public health. Sitting at the top of this pyramid are systematic reviews and meta-analyses. Why? In these disciplines, it is accepted that a systematic review and/or meta-analysis of randomised controlled trials (RCTs) is the most reliable form of evidence available. In these fields, it is commonplace to run meta-analyses because RCTs routinely collect statistical information that can be pooled using meta-analysis. In Psychology, systematic reviews have become increasingly popular but there are often issues preventing meta-analysis, namely, that psychologists use a range of research methods which can mean it is challenging to pool results. Nevertheless, adding meta-analysis to your systematic review can end up providing statistical evidence for the claims you make.

My favourite reason for running a meta-analysis is that they generate novel questions that can be tested in primary research studies. In my most recent meta-analysis, Cooke et al. (2023), we found that forming implementation intentions (if-then plans) had significantly larger effects on alcohol use in community samples compared to university samples. However, we also found that almost all community samples completed implementation intentions on paper, whereas almost all university samples completed implementation intentions online. This means we could not be sure if it was (a) the sample, (b) the mode of delivery, or (c) an interaction between sample and mode of delivery that explained these effects. Until some researchers collect data from community samples using online mode of delivery, we'll not know if they equally benefit from an alternative mode of delivery or if the mode of delivery is why implementation intentions did not reduce alcohol use in university samples. So, a tightly defined, empirically testable research question emerged from our meta-analysis. We did not set out to generate this question, it resulted from our analyses.

Alternatively, in Cooke et al. (2016), we found that adolescents reported smaller attitudes–intention and subjective norm–intention correlations compared with adults. A recent paper by Kyrrestad et al. (2020), independently confirmed that attitudes and subjective norms have small-sized effects on intentions in a large sample of Norwegian adolescents. Once again, a result of a meta-analysis set up a primary research question. While you might not change the world with your own meta-analysis, at the end of the process you will be much better informed than when you started. I think that is a good goal for any research study.

How Many Studies (Samples) Do I Need to Run a Meta-Analysis?

The simple answer to the question of how many studies you need to run a meta-analysis is two, otherwise you cannot pool results. However, I agree with Martin Hagger (Hagger, 2022) that unless both studies used robust study designs, there is not much value in pooling results together. I have been told a meta-analysis based on over 30 studies was 'premature' and received feedback on other meta-analyses saying that results would be more convincing if based on more studies. Not very helpful, having spent two years searching for studies!!!

I would say that you should aim to include effect sizes from between 30 and 40 studies (samples) for a meta-analysis, though this reflects the number of studies I have typically included in my meta-analyses rather than a definitive figure. One source of support for this claim comes from researchers using a moderator technique called meta-CART (see Chap. 14), who argue that to test moderation using this technique you need at least 40 effect sizes and that results work best with at least 120. In my experience, it's unlikely you will find 120 effect sizes, unless you are looking to update an existing meta-analysis, so, you will likely have to make do with the studies you can find. The more the better though.

Summary

In this chapter, I've introduced you to what meta-analysis is, what it involves, and why you should run a meta-analysis. In the next chapter, I'll discuss effect sizes in more detail as these are the building blocks of meta-analysis.

References

Ajzen, I. (1991). The theory of planned behavior. *Organizational Behavior and Human Decision Processes, 50*, 179–211. https://doi.org/10.1016/0749-5978(91)90020-T

Ajzen, I., & Fishbein, M. (1973). Attitudinal and normative variables as predictors of specific behaviors. *Journal of Personality and Social Psychology, 27*, 41–57.

Armitage, C. J., & Conner, M. (2001). Efficacy of the theory of planned behaviour: A meta-analytic review. *British Journal of Social Psychology, 40*(4), 471–499. https://doi.org/10.1348/014466601164939

Ashford, S., Edmunds, J., & French, D. P. (2010). What is the best way to change self-efficacy to promote lifestyle and recreational physical activity? A systematic review with meta-analysis. *British Journal of Health Psychology, 15*(2), 265–288. https://doi.org/10.1348/135910709X461752

Bandura, A. (1977). Self-efficacy: toward a unifying theory of behavioral change. *Psychological review, 84*(2), 191–215

Borenstein, M., Hedges, L. V., Higgins, J., & Rothstein, H. R. (Eds.). (2009). *Introduction to meta-analysis* (1st ed.). Wiley.

Borenstein, M., Hedges, L. V., Higgins, J., & Rothstein, H. R. (2021). *Introduction to meta-analysis* (2nd ed.). Wiley.

Chambers, C. (2017). *The seven deadly sins of psychology: A manifesto for reforming the culture of scientific practice / Chris Chambers*. Princeton University Press.

Cohen, J. (1992). A power primer. *Psychological Bulletin, 112*(1), 155–159.

Cooke, R., Dahdah, M., Norman, P., & French, D. P. (2016). How well does the theory of planned behaviour predict alcohol consumption? A systematic review and meta-analysis. *Health Psychology Review, 10*, 148–167. https://doi.org/10.1080/17437199.2014.947547

Cooke, R., McEwan, H., & Norman, P. (2023). The effect of forming implementation intentions on alcohol consumption: A systematic review and meta-analysis. *Drug and Alcohol Review, 42*, 68–80. https://doi.org/10.1111/dar.13553

Epton, T., Harris, P. R., Kane, R., van Koningsbruggen, G. M., & Sheeran, P. (2015). The impact of self-affirmation on health-behavior change: A meta-analysis. *Health Psychology, 34*(3), 187–196. https://doi.org/10.1037/hea0000116

Gollwitzer, P. M., & Sheeran, P. (2006). Implementation intentions and goal achievement: A meta-analysis of effects and processes. *Advances in Experimental Social Psychology, 38*, 69–119. https://doi.org/10.1016/S0065-2601(06)38002-1

Hagger, M. S. (2022). Meta-analysis. *International Review of Sport and Exercise Psychology, 15*(1), 120–151. https://doi.org/10.1080/1750984X.2021.1966824

Kyrrestad, H., Mabille, G., Adolfsen, F., Koposov, R., & Martinussen, M. (2020). Gender differences in alcohol onset and drinking frequency in adolescents: An application of the theory of planned behavior. *Drugs: Education, Prevention and Policy*, 1–11. https://doi.org/10.1080/09687637.2020.1865271

McEachan, R. R. C., Conner, M., Taylor, N. J., & Lawton, R. J. (2011). Prospective prediction of health-related behaviours with the Theory of Planned Behaviour: A meta-analysis. *Health Psychology Review, 5*, 97–144. https://doi.org/10.1080/17437199.2010.521684

Michie, S., Van Stralen, M. M., & West, R. (2011). The behaviour change wheel: A new method for characterising and designing behaviour change interventions. *Implementation Science, 6*(1), 42. https://doi.org/10.1186/1748-5908-6-42

Sheeran, P., Listrom, O., & Gollwitzer, P. M. (2024). The when and how of planning: Meta-analysis of the scope and components of implementation intentions in 642 tests. *European Review of Social Psychology*, 1–33. https://doi.org/10.1080/10463283.2024.2334563

Sheeran, P., & Orbell, S. (1998). Do intentions predict condom use? Metaanalysis and examination of six moderator variables. *British Journal of Social Psychology, 37*(2), 231–250. https://doi.org/10.1111/j.2044-8309.1998.tb01167.x

Identifying Your Effect Size

3

Identifying Your Effect Size

A key question to answer when writing the protocol for the systematic review that will inform your meta-analysis is "What effect size will be used to pool results from included studies?" Effect sizes are summary statistics reported in primary studies, like the correlation between two variables (r) or the effect size difference (d) between two groups in an outcome. Meta-analysis involves pooling (synthesising) effect sizes, so, until you identify your effect size, you won't be able to conduct a meta-analysis.

Part of the process of identifying your effect size is knowing what statistics go hand-in-hand with different study designs. In many papers, the study design used by researchers determines the effect size reported; observational (survey) designs usually report correlations between variables, whereas experimental (intervention/trial) designs usually report descriptive statistics (mean, standard deviation) for an outcome. The two most reported effect sizes that psychologists use in meta-analyses are correlations between variables and effect size differences in an outcome. I'll use two of my meta-analyses as examples to help you start thinking about your effect size:

- Cooke et al. (2016) is a meta-analysis of studies applying Ajzen's (1991) theory of planned behaviour to predict drinking intentions and drinking behaviour. According to the theory, attitudes, subjective norms, and perceived behavioural control should all correlate with intentions, and intentions and perceived behavioural control should both correlate with alcohol use. Researchers have mainly tested these predictions using cross-sectional tests of attitude–intention, subjective norm–intention and perceived behavioural control–intention correlations and prospective tests of intention–drinking behaviour and perceived behavioural control–drinking behaviour correlations. After systematically searching for stud-

R. Cooke, *Meta-Analysis for Psychologists*,
https://doi.org/10.1007/978-3-031-73773-2_3

ies testing the theory of planned behaviour's ability to predict drinking intentions or drinking behaviour, we extracted correlations between variables and drinking intentions or drinking behaviour before using meta-analysis to pool correlations into overall effect sizes for each theory relationship.

- Cooke et al. (2023) is a meta-analysis of studies testing the impact of forming implementation intentions—if-then plans specifying how you plan to change your behaviour (Gollwitzer, 1999)—on future alcohol consumption. Researchers used prospective designs to test effects of forming (versus not forming) implementation intentions on future behaviour. Participants report baseline performance of behaviour before being assigned to form (or not form) an implementation intention, creating intervention and control groups. The impact of forming (or not forming) implementation intentions is assessed by measuring behaviour at some point in the future, typically between one week and six weeks after forming implementation intentions. Our goal was to conduct a meta-analysis of the effect of forming implementation intentions on studies measuring alcohol use outcomes, for example, weekly drinking or heavy episodic drinking (also known as binge drinking). After systematically searching for studies that tested the effect of forming implementation intentions on alcohol use outcomes, we extracted means and standard deviations for intervention and control groups to allow us to calculate effect size differences between the two groups in alcohol use outcomes before using meta-analysis to pool effect size differences.

In the first paper, we pooled correlations to test predictions made by a theory; in the second paper, we pooled effect size differences to test an intervention; correlations and effect size differences are both effect sizes. In my experience, most psychology students are familiar with correlations, they may be less familiar with the term effect sizes and are unlikely to think of correlations as an effect size. I believe this is because most undergraduate and postgraduate psychology courses rarely describe correlations as effect sizes. This only becomes problematic when we think about other effect sizes.

A quick glance at Table 1 of Cohen's (1992) seminal paper on power shows you that there are multiple effect sizes we can use. The Pearson product moment correlation we all know and love is the second effect size in this table, identified with its letter 'r'. The table also contains other effect sizes you should be familiar with, including the chi-square goodness of fit and contingency statistic, and the f value from a one-way analysis of variance. So, you know three effect sizes already, probably without realising you do!

Cohen's table contains five other statistics that are less well known by psychologists, including the effect size difference, 'd', which is the standardised mean difference between two groups (e.g. control and intervention) on an outcome. For example, you can use means and standard deviations for weekly alcohol use reported by a control and intervention group to calculate a 'd' value.

It's probably because I like statistics that I don't fear learning about them, and it seems to me that psychology students are often reluctant to learn new approaches to analysing data due to a mix of fear of getting things wrong and a lack of confidence in what they are doing. I'll do my best in this book to help increase your confidence in using effect sizes as it is essential you understand them if you want to run a meta-analysis. The next section will take a slight detour from our focus on effect sizes to illustrate how significance is only one of three key statistical dimensions when it comes to interpreting the results of any statistical test.

Statistical Dimensions: There's More to Stats Than Significance

You can report statistical information in terms of three dimensions:

- What is the **direction** of the effect size? Is it a positive, negative, or null relationship between two variables of interest? Which group has the higher/lower mean score on the outcome you're interested in, or are the means of the two groups similar?
- What is the **magnitude** of the effect size? How large is the correlation between the two variables? How large is the difference in the outcome between two groups?
- What is the **significance** of the effect size? How likely is it that your result occurred by chance?

Twenty years of teaching UK postgraduate psychology students' statistics has shown me that completing UK undergraduate psychology statistics courses makes many postgraduate psychology students fixate on the significance of an effect size. Many students obsess over p values as a beacon of statistical knowledge—if p is under the cut-off for significance, then all is well, if not, then all is not well. I believe that statistical significance is often the least important information you can report following a statistical test, especially, if it is the only information you report. Telling me you found a significant result is way less interesting than telling me what direction the effect size shows, which is good, or the magnitude of the effect size, which is the most useful information you can report. On their own, statistical significance values tell you very little, and as we discuss later in the book, obsessing over significant results is a clear cause of publication bias (see Chap. 13).

Why do psychologists obsess over statistical significance? I think it's due to a lack of confidence in interpreting statistics, plus fear of getting things wrong, with a dash of heuristic-driven thinking. We know from social psychology that when people are uncertain, they rely on heuristics (rules of thumb) to help make decisions. Daniel Kahneman's work with Amos Tversky makes this point more eloquently than I can, so, I recommend reading his work if you want to know more (Kahneman, 2012). Applied to statistical inference, students lack confidence and are fearful of statistics, which sound like prime conditions for uncertainty. Learning the heuristic, $p < 0.05$ is good and $p > 0.05$ is bad is a great, no-fuss heuristic to get round all that fear and uncertainty. It drives me up the wall, but I understand it.

Now, with meta-analysis, you can (almost) entirely forget about significance, if you like. Pooling results using meta-analysis leads to greater focus on the direction and magnitude of effects and less emphasis on significance. I would say that the significance of a result tends to be the *least* commented dimension of a statistic in a meta-analysis. What matters more is direction and magnitude.

The Direction of an Effect Size

The direction of an effect size statistic can be reported using one of three categories: positive, negative, or null. These are reported slightly differently for correlations and effect size differences. For instance, a correlation's direction can be described as a (1) positive correlation, for example, $r = 0.45$, as attitudes towards binge drinking get more positive so do drinking intentions; (2) negative correlation, for example, $r = -0.45$, as intentions to limit binge drinking episodes increase, the frequency of binge drinking episodes decreases; or (3) null correlation, $r = 0.00$, there is no linear relationship between perceptions of control and binge drinking episodes. Alternatively, a positive effect size difference is where the intervention group do better on the outcome than the control group, for example, $d = 0.35$, intervention participants drank less alcohol than control participants, a negative effect size difference is where the control group do better on the outcome than the intervention group, for example, $d = -0.35$, control participants drank less alcohol than intervention participants, while a null effect size difference, for example, $d = 0.00$, means that control and intervention participants drank similar amounts of alcohol. The direction of an effect size is not always made explicit in psychology papers. Perhaps this is because some see it as obvious. I must admit, that outside of writing up meta-analysis results, I rarely focus on the direction of an effect size unless it is unexpected, for example, when you expect a positive correlation and find a negative one instead. Regardless of reporting of direction in primary papers, in meta-analyses, the direction of effect sizes is important to report as it helps you infer what is happening across studies. I will talk more about direction when we discuss data synthesis in Chap. 7.

The Magnitude of an Effect Size

The magnitude (size) of an effect size is the most important statistical dimension in meta-analysis; the main reason for running any meta-analysis is to precisely determine the overall effect size (sometimes called a point estimate) for your set of studies (samples). Calculating the effect size across studies enables you to speak with greater confidence about the effect size you are interested in than the authors of primary papers testing the effect size because by pooling results from multiple papers, your results are based on a meta-analysis of multiple studies (samples). This gives you greater authority about the effect size.

Magnitude is usually thought of in terms of three categories: small, medium, or large. Values for these categories differ depending on the effect size you are interested in; go back to Table 1 in Cohen (1992) to see what I mean. So, while it is true to say there are small/medium/large correlations and small/medium/large effect size differences because the ranges for these values vary, I will describe them in the sections focused on correlations and effect size differences that follow this section.

Hopefully my detour has begun to convince you of the importance of thinking beyond significance when interpreting statistics and shown the importance of thinking about the direction and magnitude of effect sizes. The next two sections introduce the two effect sizes that psychologists most commonly use in meta-analysis. I'll start with the correlation coefficient (r) because it is more familiar to psychologists, and more commonly reported in papers, than the effect size difference (d).

The Correlation Coefficient (r)—An Effect Size Familiar to Psychologists

Perhaps because my academic career began with a meta-analysis of correlations, whenever I teach a class or workshop about meta-analysis, I always begin by explaining how to run a meta-analysis of correlations. Correlations are simple to interpret in terms of direction and magnitude, which makes them a good way to start thinking about meta-analysis. An added bonus is that psychology students know about correlations, which is not something I can take for granted when I teach about meta-analysing effect size differences.

The Pearson's correlation coefficient (r) is a statistic used to test the idea there is a linear relationship between two variables. My first PhD study (Cooke & Sheeran, 2004) was a meta-analysis of correlations between variables from Ajzen's (1991) theory of planned behaviour (visit https://people.umass.edu/~aizen/ for more about this theory). I systematically searched for papers that reported correlations between attitudes and intentions, and/or correlations between intentions and behaviour, and sought to assess the impact of moderators on the size of these correlations (see Chap. 12).

Correlations are bounded statistics, meaning they fall between −1 (a perfect negative correlation) and +1 (a perfect positive correlation), with a correlation of zero (a null correlation) the middle of this range. Box 3.1 discusses why you are unlikely to see papers report perfect positive and perfect negative relationships, and quite unlikely to see papers report null relationships. Positive relationships show variables that increase in the same direction. In Cooke et al. (2016), we found positive relationships between attitudes and intentions, subjective norms and intentions, and intentions and drinking behaviour. Such results affirm the theory's proposals of linear relationships between variables and outcomes. We also found a negative relationship between perceived control and intentions, meaning those reporting *less* control over drinking had higher intentions, and a null relationship between perceived control and drinking behaviour, showing that perceptions of control were not related to drinking, across studies included in the meta-analysis. Neither result is consistent with the theory's proposals! The null relationship between perceived control and drinking behaviour led us to reflect on this result. Our answer was that results across studies were heterogeneous and were almost as dispersed as those reported by Ashford et al. (2010) (see Fig. 2.1).

Box 3.1 Why Are You Unlikely to Find Papers Reporting Perfect Negative, Perfect Positive or Null Relationships in Peer Review Journal Articles? Although it is possible for psychologists to publish papers reporting perfect negative ($r = -1$) or perfect positive ($r = 1$) correlations, it is unlikely you will find correlations like these in the published literature. One reason is that most psychologists who conduct correlational analyses are aware of the principle of multicollinearity, which is where two variables are so highly correlated they are essentially measuring the same thing. This makes the variables redundant as predictor variables in a regression model because they account for the same variance in the outcome as each other. If you include either in your model you will get similar results. Indeed, having both variables in your model reduces model fit, because you are adding two variables that account for the same variance in the outcome variable, and models fit better when predictors are (relatively) independent of one another. Statistical textbooks recommend a cut-off of $r = 0.80$ for multicollinearity when conducting regression analyses. Due to this, psychology papers rarely report results that exceed $r = 0.80$, because they know they will be criticised by reviewers for analyses that are multicollinear and hard to interpret as a result. This makes reporting perfect negative ($r = -1$) or perfect positive ($r = 1$) extremely rare in the psychological literature.

Null relationships are not necessarily as rare as perfect negative or perfect positive relations, but would appear to reflect a failure in research design—why would you want to report results of a study that shows no linear relationship between two variables you believed (before conducting the study) to be linearly related? Most of the studies I have included in meta-analyses of correlations have reported non-null relationships, although my meta-analysis of the relationships between perceived control and drinking intentions (Cooke et al., 2016) did include several studies that reported null relationships. Null relationships are likely to be rare in your literature of interest because researchers are more likely to report results that show significant linear relationships. Reporting null relationships is unlikely to help your paper get published (see Chap. 13), although the move to publish results on the Open Science Framework should help address this issue somewhat.

According to Cohen (1992), correlations can be interpreted as follows:

- Correlations between $r = 0.10$ and $r = 0.29$ are SMALL sized.
- Correlations between $r = 0.30$ and $r = 0.49$ are MEDIUM sized.
- Correlations of $r = 0.50$ or higher are LARGE sized.

It is worth noting that the sign (+ or −) before your correlation makes no difference to the magnitude of the correlation; correlations of −0.20 and 0.20 are both small sized. Box 3.2 provides an example of how to interpret a correlation from a primary study to show how to work out the direction and magnitude of individual correlations.

Often, the result reported in Box 3.2 would be used to inform further primary studies. For instance, you might want to increase physical activity intentions and believe that if you make attitudes more positive, you will increase intentions—this reasoning underlies Ajzen's (1991) theory of planned behaviour and other health psychology models of behaviour. So you design an intervention providing information to make physical activity attitudes more positive. Alternatively, the result could be the first step of a meta-analysis, a secondary study. By computing the correlation, you've taken your first step towards conducting a meta-analysis of studies that correlate physical activity attitudes with physical activity intentions. You have your first effect size needed for a meta-analysis, that is, the correlation $r = 0.35$. Your next step would be to systematically search for similar correlations reported by other researchers in academic journals, grey literature, and open science portals like the Open Science Framework (see Chap. 4). After completing the search, you identify included studies, extract the correlations and sample sizes (see Chap. 5), quality-appraise studies (see Chap. 6) before pooling results using meta-analysis (see Chap. 7).

▶ **Box 3.2 The Magnitude of a Correlation** Imagine running a study where you send a questionnaire to a sample of office employees (aged 25–35) to measure their physical activity attitudes (i.e. whether people view physical activity positively or negatively) and physical activity intentions (i.e. whether people intend or not to be physically active). You use this data to compute a correlation between physical activity attitudes and intentions. Let's imagine the correlation comes out as $r = 0.35$. This is a positive correlation, that is, as attitudes towards physical activity become more positive, so do intentions to be physically active. The magnitude of the correlation can be inferred using Cohen's (1992) guidelines reported above. In this case, it is a medium-sized correlation because $r = 0.35$ falls between $r = 0.30$ and $r = 0.49$. So, using our data, we can infer that physical activity attitudes have a medium-sized, positive, correlation with physical activity intentions.

The aim of this section was to outline how to interpret the direction and magnitude of correlations—the same process for interpreting a single correlation in terms of direction and size is used when interpreting a correlational meta-analysis. Once you have computed your sample-weighted average correlation, you interpret this with reference to Cohen's (1992) guidelines covered on the previous page. Thus, how you interpret a correlation from a single paper is identical to how you interpret the result of a meta-analysis of correlations (see Chap. 7). Having covered a statistic you are familiar with I'll next move on to one you are probably less familiar with—the effect size difference (d).

The Effect Size Difference (d)—An Effect Size Less Familiar to Psychologists

After I finish teaching postgraduate students about meta-analysis of correlations, I move on to explain meta-analysis of effect size differences. I believe that teaching students about meta-analysis of effect size differences is more conceptually challenging than teaching about meta-analysis of correlations. In part, this is because I am usually teaching students about a statistic they are unfamiliar with. This means I must explain what an effect size difference is, and how to calculate it, before I can explain how you run a meta-analysis of effect size differences. Nevertheless, it is well worth assimilating this knowledge because the methodology that underpins effect size differences, experimental designs, allow for much greater confidence in interpretation of findings than correlational designs. Of course, psychologists are interested in both methods, which is why I cover both in this book.

The effect size difference (d) is the standardised mean difference in an outcome (e.g. physical activity, drinking behaviour, quality of life, educational achievement) between two groups, (e.g. an intervention [experimental] group and a control group). For example, we might want to know if physical activity is higher in a group that received a psychologically informed intervention compared to a control group who did not receive the intervention. The effect size difference allows us to assess the extent of the difference between the two groups in the outcome, while controlling for differences in dispersion of data points in the two groups. Standardising the mean differences for each effect size allows you to pool results from studies that have used different scales/measures to assess an outcome.

Effect size differences can help you to quickly assess the impact of an intervention on an outcome of interest. For example, as I noted at the start of the chapter, we published a meta-analysis of effect size differences to estimate the pooled effect of forming versus not forming implementation intentions on alcohol consumption (Cooke et al., 2023). We found that while there was a positive, small, significant effect size difference of forming implementation intentions on weekly drinking ($d = -0.16$) there was a null effect size difference of forming implementation intentions on heavy episodic drinking ($d = 0.00$). Results show forming implementation intentions is effective at reducing weekly drinking but has no effect on heavy episodic drinking.

Effect size differences are unbounded statistics, meaning they can be as large or small as you can imagine. In my experience, effect size differences for psychology studies typically fall between $-0.50 < d < +0.50$. Like correlations, the mid-point of the range of possible values for effect size differences is $d = 0.00$, that is, there is no difference in the outcome between the two groups. This is called a null effect size difference. Like correlations, we can talk about positive effect size differences and negative effect size differences, but, because effect size differences are unbounded there is no such thing as a perfect positive or perfect negative effect size difference. A positive effect size difference usually means intervention participants have performed better on the outcome than control participants, for example, $d = 0.35$, could mean intervention participants self-reporting more physical activity three months after receiving the intervention compared to control participants. A negative effect size difference often means that scores on the outcome are **better** in the control group than the intervention group, for example, $d = -0.35$, could mean control participants self-reporting more physical activity three months after receiving the intervention compared to intervention participants. This may not be expected, but it is possible—maybe control participants were offered a free gym membership during the study.

Unlike correlations, where the sign almost always means the same direction, with effect size differences the sign depends on the order in which **you** enter the mean values for the two groups. For example, if you hypothesise there will be a positive effect size difference on physical activity of receiving the intervention, you are saying you expect that intervention participants will increase their physical activity at follow-up more than control participants. If this is the case, enter your intervention mean first which has the effect of producing a positive result because the control mean will be subtracted from the intervention mean like this:

1. Intervention group physical activity (M)—Control group physical activity (M).
2. 15.00–10.00 = 5.00 (i.e. the mean difference between the groups).
3. Divide this value by the pooled standard deviation.
4. You now have your standardised mean difference also known as the effect size difference (d) which has a positive direction.

There are also times when you expect to calculate negative effect size differences, for example, if you hypothesise a greater reduction in an outcome in the intervention group than the control (e.g. the intervention group report drinking less alcohol than the control group). For example, in Cooke et al. (2023) we expected the effect of the intervention was to reduce drinking behaviour more in participants who formed implementation intentions. Here is an example of what happens when you do this:

1. Intervention group alcohol use (M)—Control group alcohol use (M).
2. 15.00–25.00 = −10.00 (this is the mean difference between the groups).
3. Divide this value by the pooled standard deviation.
4. You now have your standardised mean difference also known as the effect size difference (d) which has a negative direction.

The key is to decide prior to conducting your meta-analysis which direction you want to compute effect size differences when you report results and then set up your analysis to be consistent when conducting the meta-analysis. Always ensure you enter data in a consistent way otherwise it will be hard to interpret your meta-analysis.

Cohen's (1992) guidelines for interpreting effect size differences are as follows:

- Effect size differences between $d = 0.20$ and $d = 0.49$ are SMALL sized.
- Effect size differences between $d = 0.50$ and $d = 0.79$ are MEDIUM sized.
- Effect size differences of $d = 0.80$ or higher are LARGE sized.

It is worth noting that the sign (+ or −) before your effect size difference makes no difference to the magnitude of the effect size difference; $d = -0.30$ and $d = 0.30$ are both small sized. However, as discussed above, be mindful of how you decided to calculate your effect size differences because unlike correlations, the sign (+ or −) you decide on can affect the direction you report (see above). Box 3.3 provides an example of how you can interpret the direction and size of an individual effect size difference from a primary study.

Box 3.3 provides lots of useful information. We can see that the intervention had a positive effect on intentions because $d = 0.25$; after receiving the intervention, people in the intervention group reported higher physical activity intentions compared to people in the control group. We can also see the effect size difference is small sized, meaning that our researcher's intervention did not produce large changes in intentions. This might make our researcher decide they need to refine their intervention to make it more effective.

Box 3.3 The Magnitude of an Effect Size Difference Following on from our earlier example in Box 3.2, let's assume that our researcher decided to deliver an intervention to make physical activity attitudes more positive to increase physical activity intentions among our sample of office workers. They develop an intervention to highlight the benefits of physical activity and deliver it to office workers who work for one company A based on the 1st floor of a high-rise building. These workers are labelled the intervention group and asked to report their attitudes and intentions before receiving the intervention and at follow-up, three months later. Our researcher also asks workers from company B, who are also based on the 1st floor, to report their attitudes and intentions, but these workers do not receive the intervention and labelled the control group. Our researcher computes the effect size difference in intentions between intervention and control group participants, following the intervention, to be $d = 0.25$.

The result from Box 3.3 could also provide the start of a meta-analysis, including this effect size difference alongside other published examples of interventions targeting physical activity intentions. Your next step would be to systematically search for studies that also test the effects of interventions aiming to change intentions by making attitudes towards physical activity more positive published in academic journals, grey literature, and open science portals like the Open Science Framework (see Chap. 4). After completing the search, you identify included studies, extract the means, standard deviations, and sample sizes (see Chap. 5) for both intervention and control groups, quality-appraise the studies (see Chap. 6) before pooling the results using meta-analysis (see Chap. 7).

The aim of this section was to outline how to interpret the direction and magnitude of effect size differences—the same process for interpreting a single effect size difference in terms of direction and size is used when interpreting a meta-analysis of effect size differences. Once you have your sample-weighted average effect size difference, you interpret this with reference to Cohen's (1992) guidelines mentioned above. Thus, how you interpret an effect size difference from a single paper is identical to how you interpret the result of a meta-analysis of effect size differences (see Chap. 7). I will end this section by covering a common error in using Cohen's guidelines.

A Common Error in Using Cohen's Guidelines to Interpret Meta-Analytic Results

I want to share a common error psychology postgraduate students made when I assessed their knowledge of Cohen's guidelines for correlations and effect size differences. This error relates to the fact that the value 0.50 means different things for correlations and effect size differences. $r = 0.5$ is a large-sized correlation, whereas $d = 0.5$ is a medium effect size difference. It's a common error to make but you must try and avoid it otherwise you will be overselling your effect size difference. The following phrase might help—it's much easier in psychology to find a large correlation than a large effect size difference…

The above statement is based on an academic lifetime of reading and reviewing meta-analyses written by psychologists. We typically find small (Black et al., 2016; Cooke et al., 2023; Newby et al., 2021) or medium (Gollwitzer & Sheeran, 2006) effect size differences of psychological interventions. I suspect there are multiple reasons for this, including, the challenge of changing human behaviour, and in particular, uncertainty that using the same intervention methods will work for all people. I've not seen much evidence that when it comes to psychological interventions 'one size fits all'. I'm making you aware of this point to provide a warning that if you find that most of the effect size differences in your meta-analysis are large-sized you might want to check your calculations ☺.

Summary

The goal of this chapter was to introduce you to effect sizes, clarifying information you already know about correlations and helping introduce effect size differences. Because effect sizes are so instrumental to understanding meta-analysis, we will return to them throughout the book. You may want to revisit the material covered in this chapter as it often takes me a few go's reading through material on new statistical information for the penny to fully drop. The tasks on the next page should also help you to develop your knowledge and confidence about effect sizes.

Having introduced effect sizes in this chapter, we are next going to move on to cover systematic review essentials in Chap. 4, followed by chapters on data extraction (Chap. 5), quality appraisal (Chap. 6), and data synthesis (Chap. 7).

Tasks

Complete these tasks to reinforce your learning of the principles covered in this chapter.

1. What are the three statistical dimensions you can use to interpret the result of a statistical test?
2. A correlation of $r = 0.55$ is what magnitude according to Cohen's (1992) guidelines?
3. You conduct a meta-analysis of studies assessing the magnitude of the correlation between intentions and physical activity, which produces a result of $r = 0.38$. Describe this effect size in terms of direction and magnitude.
4. An effect size difference of $d = 0.55$ is what magnitude according to Cohen's (1992) guidelines?
5. You conduct a meta-analysis of studies testing the impact of receiving a goal-setting intervention to increase physical activity. The meta-analysis produces a value of $d = 0.35$. Describe this effect size in terms of direction and magnitude.
6. Is it easier to find a large-sized correlation or a large-sized effect size difference?

References

Ajzen, I. (1991). The theory of planned behavior. *Organizational Behavior and Human Decision Processes, 50*, 179–211. https://doi.org/10.1016/0749-5978(91)90020-T

Ashford, S., Edmunds, J., & French, D. P. (2010). What is the best way to change self-efficacy to promote lifestyle and recreational physical activity? A systematic review with meta-analysis. *British Journal of Health Psychology, 15*(2), 265–288. https://doi.org/10.1348/135910709X461752

Black, N., Mullan, B., & Sharpe, L. (2016). Computer-delivered interventions for reducing alcohol consumption: Meta-analysis and meta-regression using behaviour change techniques and theory. *Health Psychology Review, 10*, 341–357. https://doi.org/10.1080/17437199.2016.1168268

Cohen, J. (1992). A power primer. *Psychological Bulletin, 112*(1), 155–159.

Cooke, R., Dahdah, M., Norman, P., & French, D. P. (2016). How well does the theory of planned behaviour predict alcohol consumption? A systematic review and meta-analysis. *Health Psychology Review, 10*, 148–167. https://doi.org/10.1080/17437199.2014.947547

Cooke, R., McEwan, H., & Norman, P. (2023). The effect of forming implementation intentions on alcohol consumption: A systematic review and meta-analysis. *Drug and Alcohol Review, 42*, 68–80. https://doi.org/10.1111/dar.13553

Cooke, R., & Sheeran, P. (2004). Moderation of cognition-intention and cognition-behaviour relations: A meta-analysis of properties of variables from the theory of planned behaviour. *The British Journal of Social Psychology, 43*(Pt 2), 159–186. https://doi.org/10.1348/0144666041501688

Gollwitzer, P. M. (1999). Implementation intentions: Strong effects of simple plans. *American Psychologist, 54*(7), 493–503. https://doi.org/10.1037/0003-066X.54.7.493

Gollwitzer, P. M., & Sheeran, P. (2006). Implementation intentions and goal achievement: A meta-analysis of effects and processes. *Advances in Experimental Social Psychology, 38*, 69–119. https://doi.org/10.1016/S0065-2601(06)38002-1

Kahneman, D. (2012). *Thinking, fast and slow*. Penguin Books.

Newby, K., Teah, G., Cooke, R., Li, X., Brown, K., Salisbury-Finch, B., Kwah, K., Bartle, N., Curtis, K., Fulton, E., Parsons, J., Dusseldorp, E., & Williams, S. L. (2021). Do automated digital health behaviour change interventions have a positive effect on self-efficacy? A systematic review and meta-analysis. *Health Psychology Review, 15*(1), 140–158. https://doi.org/10.1080/17437199.2019.1705873

Part II

Preparing to Conduct a Meta-Analysis

Systematic Review Essentials 4

Systematic Review Essentials

All meta-analyses should be based on the results of a systematic review of the literature, which means it is important I cover some essential information about what conducting a systematic review involves. It is beyond the scope of this book to do more than introduce these ideas. For more information on systematic reviewing, I recommend reading one of the many excellent books on this topic (e.g. Boland et al., 2017). My focus in this chapter and the remainder of this section of the book (i.e. Chaps. 5, 6 and 7) is to provide a brief guide to systematic reviewing when conducting a meta-analysis. This chapter will emphasise the similarities between meta-analysis and systematic reviewing, with Chaps. 5, 6 and 7 focusing on differences between meta-analysis and systematic reviewing when thinking about Data Extraction (Chap. 5) Quality Appraisal (Chap. 6) and Data Synthesis (Chap. 7).

When I teach postgraduate psychology students about systematic reviewing, I begin by outlining the six steps I follow when conducting a systematic review:

1. Specifying your review question
2. Defining your inclusion criteria
3. Stating your search strategy
4. Data extraction
5. Quality appraisal
6. Data synthesis

To complete a meta-analysis, you also need to follow these steps, although how you complete them sometimes differs between meta-analysis and systematic reviewing. The main aim of this chapter is to talk you through the first three steps as they apply to conducting a meta-analysis. While much of this advice also applies to conducting a systematic review, I wanted to give explicit examples for those running a

R. Cooke, *Meta-Analysis for Psychologists*,
https://doi.org/10.1007/978-3-031-73773-2_4

meta-analysis following these steps. If you are familiar with these steps, you are welcome to head to Chap. 5 on Data Extraction.

Step 1. Specifying Your Review Question

As is the case with any research study, it is important to specify a research question in advance of conducting the study. For meta-analyses (and systematic reviews) I think of these as review questions, which are the equivalent of research questions in primary papers when you are conducting a secondary analysis. Clearly specifying your review question helps you to screen out irrelevant papers. Below are review questions my meta-analyses of correlations:

- Cooke and Sheeran (2004) 'The main aim of the present study is to provide the first quantitative review of the properties of cognitions as moderators of cognition-intention and cognition-behaviour relations.'
- Cooke and French (2008) 'The present study examines the strength of five relationships within the TRA/TPB—attitude-intention, subjective norm-intention, PBC-intention, intention-behaviour, PBC-behaviour—in the context of individuals attending a health screening programme'.
- Cooke et al. (2016). 'The present study examines the size of nine relationships within the TPB in the context of alcohol consumption: attitude-intention, subjective norm-intention, PBC-intention, SE-intention, PC-intention, intention-behaviour, PBC-behaviour, SE-behaviour, PC-behaviour'.

As you can see, there is some consistency in how these questions are phrased—all three refer to relations or relationships, explicitly telling the reader we meta-analysed correlations, because correlations are used to test relationships between variables. The 2008 and 2016 metas (short for meta-analysis) both specify a behaviour type, health screening programme, alcohol consumption, respectively, to narrow the focus of the meta-analysis. As the aim of the 2004 meta was to meta-analyse properties of cognition (e.g. how accessible attitudes were in memory, how stable intentions were over time) as moderators of cognition–intention (e.g. attitude–intention) and cognition–behaviour (intention–behaviour) relations, we did not specify a behaviour type in this question. We wanted to include all studies we could find.

Reflecting on these questions, when constructing a review question for a correlational meta-analysis, I would include the word relation or relationship or association in the question. You may also specify a behaviour type(s) for correlations you are interested in, like in the 2008 and 2016 papers. If you are interested in meta-analysing results from studies testing a theory, you could mention this in the question, like we did in the 2008 meta.

Below are examples of review questions from meta-analyses of experimental studies I authored or co-authored:

- Newby et al. (2021). 'What is the overall effect of digital automated behaviour change interventions on self-efficacy?'
- Cooke et al. (2023). 'The primary aim of the present systematic review and meta-analysis is to estimate the effect of forming implementation intentions on weekly alcohol consumption'.

Both questions mention 'the effect of…' something which speaks to including data from studies testing an experimental manipulation or evaluating an intervention designed to cause a change in an outcome of interest, which meta-analysts will recognise as a meta of effect size differences (see Chap. 3). Both questions mention an intervention type: digital automated behaviour change; implementation intentions. A difference between the questions is in the focus (or not) on a behaviour type.

These questions broadly map onto the PICO (Population, Intervention, Comparator, Outcome) framework (described in more detail in 'Step 2. Defining your inclusion criteria'). They both refer to an Intervention type (digital behaviour change; implementation intentions) and an Outcome (self-efficacy; alcohol consumption). Moreover, intervention studies often include a Comparator (control/comparison) group. No Population though! PICO was developed for studies testing RCTs, which by design have an Intervention group, at least one Comparator (control/comparison) group, an Outcome, and often, a target Population. I think PICO is more helpful for psychologists running meta-analyses of effect size differences than meta-analyses of correlations for several reasons, including - meta-analyses of correlations including data from samples who did not receive an intervention (or control) material, and there not being an obvious outcome, as, you are interested in pooling results from a correlation not an effect size difference based on an outcome. This is not to say you cannot use PICO in crafting correlational meta-analysis questions, only that it is not easy to do so.

How Many Review Questions Should I Specify?

Psychologists conducting meta-analysis often want to answer multiple questions. The above review questions are all examples of main questions and were listed first in the papers, signifying their importance. A common second review question is to specify moderators (see Chap. 12) that you think might affect heterogeneity between studies in the overall effect size. Here're some examples from the papers I have already introduced:

- Cooke et al. (2016). 'The second aim is to assess the extent to which several *moderator* variables affect the size of TPB relationships: (a) pattern of consumption, (b) gender of participants and (c) age of participants'.
- Newby et al. (2021). 'Does the overall effect of automated digital behaviour change interventions on self-efficacy vary as a function of *the behaviour* being addressed?'

- Cooke et al. (2023). 'The secondary aim is to investigate the impact of sample type, mode of delivery, intervention format and time frame as *moderators* of effect size differences'.

In each case, we are telling the reader we believe that the effect sizes of included studies may differ due to a moderator variable(s) and that we need to test these effects. This is common practice in meta-analysis, as, it is almost always the case that there is significant heterogeneity in effect sizes between studies in the overall effect size. When completing pre-registration of the systematic review that informs your meta-analysis, for example, by pre-registering your review protocol with PROSPERO, it is a good idea to mention moderators too. I will discuss pre-registration at the end of this chapter.

Step 2. Defining Your Inclusion Criteria

Defining your inclusion criteria is an important step of a systematic review because it determines which studies will be included and which excluded. In general, meta-analyses tend to be more exclusive than systematic reviews. One reason for this is that meta-analysis requires authors to report statistical information to meet inclusion criteria, whereas systematic reviews often do not. This means you may end up excluding papers from a meta-analysis that you would include in a systematic review on the same topic. The meta-analyses I have first-authored always include a criterion about reporting statistical information. For example, Cooke et al.'s (2016) fourth inclusion criterion is

- 'A bivariate statistical relationship between TPB constructs and intention had to be retrievable, either from the paper or upon request from the authors'.

Equivalently, Cooke et al.'s (2023) fourth criterion is

- 'Studies had to report the sample size for both control and intervention groups and the mean and SD (standard deviation) for the outcome variable(s)…to allow for calculation of the effect size difference (d)'.

Specifying a statistical inclusion criterion tells the reader that a lack of statistical information is grounds to exclude a study from a meta-analysis. When statistical information is not reported in the paper that meets all other inclusion criteria, my next step is to email the authors to request the information. I first had to do this when completing Cooke and Sheeran (2004) and while it felt quite intimidating as a PhD student to contact academics about their work, my experience of doing so has been overwhelmingly positive. In one case, an author went and dug out data from a set of old files! In other cases, authors report how happy they are that someone has shown interest in their research—I'm always delighted to be asked to provide data from one of my studies and do my best to respond to all requests I get.

Sometimes, the information is not available, however. A glance at the bottom of Fig. 1.1 in Newby et al. (2021) shows that we excluded four papers due to insufficient statistical information. We attempted to obtain the information from the study authors but did not receive responses to our requests. If your goal is to conduct a meta-analysis, you need data to include in the study; no data = no inclusion.

Other inclusion criteria in meta-analyses refer to study design, sampling, or outcome measures. In a meta-analysis of effect size differences, it is common to refer to study design issues in your inclusion criteria: In Cooke et al. (2023), we stated that studies must have a control (comparison) group as well as a group that formed implementation intentions; in Newby et al. (2021), we only included studies that used randomised controlled trial or quasi-randomised controlled trial designs. Newby et al. (2021) also specified the need for studies to recruit general population/non-clinical samples. In terms of outcome measures, Cooke et al. (2023) specified that the outcome, alcohol consumption, had to be measured in terms of either weekly drinking or heavy episodic drinking episodes (aka binge drinking).

A common criterion is to limit inclusion of studies where results are not reported in English. This is typically a pragmatic criterion but can limit the number of papers you include in your meta-analysis, and you should not feel bound to follow this criterion, particularly if you are conducting the meta-analysis as part of a team, whose members may be fluent in other languages. I'd say it's about being pragmatic and working out what is possible to achieve given the resources available to you. Another criterion that is sometimes used in a meta-analysis is to specify a time limit for publication, such as the last five years or the last ten years. While there are justifiable concerns that older publications may use weaker study designs, that does not strike me as good grounds to exclude them. You can use quality appraisal to assess the papers (see Chap. 6). I've had various conversations about restricting the publication range to reduce the number of papers to screen. This is not good practice! If you want fewer studies to screen, you need a better search strategy (see below). A better use of time limits is when some change has taken place to practise, for example, change in definitions for mental health issues, which means that older papers are no longer relevant. You may also justify your time frame being restricted IF a previous meta-analysis has covered literature up to a certain date, arguing that your meta covers more recent work.

How Many Inclusion Criteria Should I Have in a Meta-Analysis?

The meta-analyses I have authored or co-authored have had between three and six inclusion criteria, apart from my first (Cooke & Sheeran, 2004). There is one criterion I almost always use: all my metas refer to measurement of an outcome (Cooke et al., 2023; Newby et al., 2021) or a relationship between two variables (Cooke & French 2008; Cooke & Sheeran, 2004; Cooke et al., 2016). I would argue that this will be the case with your meta-analysis too—I find it hard to imagine how you could conduct a meta-analysis without referring to measurement in the inclusion criteria because measurement, either of outcomes measured following exposure to an experimental manipulation or an intervention, or of a correlation between two variables, are the units of analysis for the meta-analysis. Without these, you cannot run a meta-analysis.

Other criterion are only appropriate to use in particular meta-analyses; in Newby et al. (2021), we focused on non-clinical samples, while in Birdi et al. (2020), the focus was on patients with atopic dermatitis. These are the only two meta-analyses I've been involved with that have specified a population as an inclusion criterion. Alternatively, in Cooke and French (2008), we wanted to include papers that tested either the theory of reasoned action (Ajzen & Fishbein, 1973) or the theory of planned behaviour (Ajzen, 1991), so we included a criterion about papers reporting results testing theoretical relationships. You may not have something that specific in your meta, but if you do, then include it because it will help you to exclude less relevant studies when screening. One of the reasons that meta-analyses typically contain fewer studies than systematic reviews is that we specify criteria that exclude papers.

A Brief Section on PICO

I use the Table 4.1 when introducing PICO and acknowledge that it can be a really useful way to think about a systematic review, especially if you are reviewing a literature that uses RCTs or experiments, to evaluate effects on an outcome.

I also think that PICO can be useful for meta-analyses of experimental/intervention studies, with a slight modification. I teach my students that I prefer PICOS to PICO because when I conduct systematic reviews, it is likely there will be heterogeneity in study designs. In PICO, it is assumed that all studies will use an RCT study design, which makes sense if you are looking at things from a public health perspective—why would you want to include studies that use weaker study designs when you are evaluating important public health issues? To the humble psychologist, however, we must accept that there aren't likely to be as many RCTs in our field. Instead, we are likely to find a range of different study designs, including factorial designs with two or more groups (control, experimental/intervention), pre-post designs, quasi-experiments, and some RCTs. We are also unlikely to have

Table 4.1 PICO categories

PICO tool	Area	Definition
P	Population	Population of interest, e.g., cancer patients, schoolchildren, young adults, middle-aged drinkers
I	Intervention	Intervention type, e.g., implementation intentions, digital behaviour change, motivational interviewing, drinking refusal skills
C	Comparator	Comparison group, e.g., control group, matched control, other intervention group
O	Outcome	Outcome, e.g., quality of life, self-efficacy, alcohol consumption, resilience, vaccine uptake

sufficient papers in our meta-analysis to be picky about excluding papers due to study design. Where I think PICO can be helpful is when you are thinking about your search terms (see next section) because it helps you make explicit the terms, phrases, objects, concepts, et cetera you are interested in searching for and gets you thinking about what you want to include versus what you want to exclude.

Without wishing to deny the benefits of using PICO when conducting meta-analyses of experimental designs or interventions, I do not believe that PICO is always helpful when conducting meta-analysis for two reasons. First, PICO categories may not be relevant to your meta-analysis; as noted above, only Birdi et al. (2020) and Newby et al. (2021) mentioned Population as an inclusion criterion in my meta-analyses. Most of my meta-analyses are in areas where there are relatively few studies, so, the need to exclude papers based on population is not that important. Similarly, if you are conducting a meta-analysis of correlational studies, then there is no Intervention or Comparator. For correlational meta-analyses, there is not really an Outcome either, because you are interested in the correlation between an outcome and a predictor (or sometimes, two predictors). Second, PICO makes no reference to theories. This likely reflects disciplinary differences between psychologists (who love a theory) and medicine/public health (who appear less in love with theory). In Cooke and French (2008) and Cooke et al. (2016), we used theory to limit our search as we were only interested in papers that tested theoretical predictions. This may be a health/social psychology thing, as there are a lot of reviews of this type (Hagger et al., 2017; Todd et al., 2016; van Lettow et al., 2016), but it does limit the utility of PICO for certain meta-analyses of psychological studies.

Step 3. Stating Your Search Strategy

A search strategy is your search terms plus your search sources. Ideally, your strategy should use terms that mainly access relevant papers for your meta-analysis, but in reality, you often end up with a lot of irrelevant studies. I'll start by discussing search sources and then move on to search terms.

Search Sources

Search sources are the places you search to identify papers to include in your meta-analysis, for example, bibliographic databases, journals, websites that publish reports, et cetera. The choice of sources determines what you will find. Most systematic reviews and meta-analyses search from a rather restrictive pool of databases, with apparently little justification or rationale for this decision. I suspect that many researchers do what I do which is to use databases we are familiar with or those that have been used in previously published review articles. There is some merit in this idea, because to my knowledge no one has set down any criteria for which databases one should search or how many one should search. Without criteria, researchers tend to do what they think makes sense, with an eye to existing papers as a guide.

Looking back over my meta-analyses, I searched between two and six databases. I always searched Web of Science, because this was the database I was taught how to use during my PhD. Web of Science always seemed to produce a set of relevant results from the psychological literature. Since Cooke and French (2008), I've also always searched PubMed (sometimes as part of MEDLINE). This reflects my move from social to health psychology; PubMed is a good journal for checking medicine and public health journals and is free to use because it is maintained by the National Institute for Health in the USA. Searching PubMed and Web of Science using the same search terms is a good way to see what two databases, which index different journals return in response. If, after your search, you find a paper in both databases then you know they both index that journal. If you find a relevant reference in one but not the other database, you can be sure that both databases don't index that journal. This is a key reason to search more than one database. If you only search one, you might miss relevant papers for your meta.

In addition to these two mainstays of my search sources, I often searched another database that I was confident would index psychology articles, like PsychArticles or PsychInfo. This was done to check that my Web of Science results were not missing relevant studies published in journals not indexed by Web of Science. I've also contributed to searches where we have used Scopus, and that seems like a good option for psychologists, if you don't have access to Web of Science. In Cooke et al. (2023), because we were searching for intervention studies, I also searched the Cochrane database. If you are doing a meta-analysis of effect size differences, it is worth searching the Cochrane database to ensure someone else has not already done the meta you are planning to do! Other databases that might be relevant for **your** meta-analysis include CINAHL (a database of nursing research), EMBASE (a database of medical research, that requires a subscription). There are probably other databases relevant for educational, organisational, forensic, and other psychological subdisciplines, but, as I've not done reviews in these areas, I do not know what they are.

I have also searched Google Scholar when conducting a meta-analysis and while I think it is ok to include this as one of several search sources, I would not exclusively search Google Scholar when conducting your search because it is unclear whether all papers have been peer reviewed. Nevertheless, searching Google Scholar can identify papers missed by other databases, and indexes citations in languages other than English, so it is worth considering as one of your sources.

In Cooke and Sheeran (2004) and Cooke et al. (2023), I also searched grey literature, also known as unpublished literature. In both cases, I searched databases that index PhD theses and this was done to ensure that I found as many papers as possible because there was a lack of research studies. In the UK and Ireland, the database of all PhD theses is called EThOS. It is open access, so feel free to search for completeness or if you find a lack of papers.

Sometimes, I am asked how many sources should I search? I have seen some reviews where teams have searched more than ten databases, which seems excessive to me. Searching is a resource-intensive activity and while searching ten databases seems better than searching four or five, my thought on this is how many additional, unique, papers does searching the additional five databases generate (and is it worth doing)? The law of diminishing returns would suggest you are better off searching fewer databases that are likely to contain the most relevant studies for your meta-analysis.

I'll end with some advice about which sources to search. First, always search a source that indexes the psychological literature: Scopus, Web of Science, or any database with the word Psych in the title are good options to meet this criterion. Second, always search a source that indexes a related, but relevant, area. As a Health Psychologist, PubMed fulfils this criterion for me. If you are an educational (or developmental) psychologist, then look for databases of educational research to search. If you are unsure how to find these, look at published meta-analyses or systematic reviews from your area to see which databases were searched. Third, always search at least two databases—this protects you against missing papers due to indexing issues with the databases. No database indexes all journals. Finally, think carefully about whether to search the grey literature or not. If you are conducting a search for studies on a popular topic, for example, interventions to promote healthy eating in children, you will likely find enough studies for a meta-analysis without searching the grey literature. Similarly, if you are interested in RCTs, you are unlikely to find too many of these in the grey literature. If, on the other hand, you are searching for studies on more obscure topics, like in Cooke and Sheeran (2004), it makes sense to look at the grey literature, especially PhD theses, because this might help increase your set of studies. I think the key question is to ask yourself 'Why should I search the grey literature?' and if you can come up with any plausible answer, then go ahead and search!

Search Terms

Search terms are the words or phrases used to identify relevant studies when searching an electronic database. While your set of search terms can end up being really lengthy, as you come up with all the synonyms you can think of, I usually generate my list of terms by going back to the review question. Let's use Cooke and French (2008) as an example. Here's the review question again:

- Review Question 'The present study examines the strength of five relationships within the TRA/TPB—attitude-intention, subjective norm-intention, PBC-intention, intention-behaviour, PBC-behaviour—in the context of individuals attending a health screening programme.'

  And here are the search terms

- Search Terms
- 'theory of reasoned action', 'theory of planned behavio*[1]', 'screening', mammograph', 'cervical', 'health check/screening' and 'attend'.

[1]The asterisk is known as a wildcard. It means that when searching any paper that contains the letters before the * will be included in the search list regardless of what follows. In this case, we inserted the * because we wanted to make sure our output contained papers using both the English

This set of search terms probably seems very short, but it captures the essentials of the review question—we searched for papers on the theory of reasoned action and theory of planned behaviour in screening contexts. Other terms (mammograph, cervical, health check/screening) were included in case a more specific type of screening (e.g. cervical) was mentioned in the abstract. Because we were interested in papers that tested theories, we ended up with a small set of search terms. If either theory was not mentioned in the abstract, then we excluded the paper. This is an example of how jargon can be advantageous. You can also see we did not make any reference to study type in our search terms. As most studies testing these theories used correlational designs, there was no need to specify a design. Please note this may not be the case with your meta-analysis, so, be mindful of study design when thinking about your own search terms.

Let's next look at the review question and search terms for Cooke et al. (2023):

- Review Question: 'The primary aim of the present systematic review and meta-analysis is to estimate the effect of forming implementation intentions on weekly alcohol consumption.'
- Search Terms
- 'implementation intentions', 'alcohol', 'binge drink*'.

Even fewer search terms than the ones above!!! Once again, we took advantage of jargon, specifically, the phrase implementation intentions. We were able to exclude many papers because they did not mention implementation intentions. The meta-analyses I have co-authored (Birdi et al., 2020; Newby et al., 2021), have typically used broader search terms, so, I am not saying you must be as minimalist as I am. However, there can be a cost to having too many search terms; finding 1000s (or 10,000s) of irrelevant papers. I've read abstracts where researchers report results of a systematic review that screened 30,000 or 40,000 results. That seems wasteful to me, especially as these comprehensive reviews have not yielded many more papers for inclusion than my approach. There is a balance to strike between being comprehensive in your searching, by using broad terms that capture all the relevant papers but also a lot of irrelevant papers, and more specific searching that may miss a few relevant papers but also excludes most of the irrelevant papers you would have excluded anyway. In a meta-analysis, I would always favour more specific search terms because your goal is to pool results testing an effect size. Unless papers report a test of a specific effect size, you are probably not going to be able to include the paper.

Another thing to bear in mind when doing a meta-analysis, as opposed to a systematic review, is that the meta-analysis requires the study to report statistical information to be included, whereas a systematic review does not. Based on my experience of searching for papers to include in meta-analyses, you should expect to find a relatively small pool of studies to full-text screen. I typically find between

and American spellings of the word behaviour (behaviour, behavior). Locating the * after the o, the last letter than is common to both spellings, achieved that aim.

150 and 300 papers to screen. I would say, if you have more than 1000 hits after removing duplications for a *meta-analysis*, you should probably go back to your search terms and see if there is a way to reduce this number. While I think it's reasonable to have more than 1000 hits for a systematic review, I would be wary of screening more than 1000 hits for a meta-analysis because I think it's highly unlikely you will find sufficient papers have included the statistical information needed for your meta. To quote Hagger et al.'s exceptionally impressive meta-analysis of the common sense model of illness (2017):

> *The literature research identified 333 articles that met inclusion criteria on initial screening...A substantial proportion of eligible articles (k = 172) did report the necessary data for analysis.*

This meta-analysis is an update of a previously published meta-analysis on the same model (Hagger & Orbell, 2003), which likely explains why the authors found so many relevant papers. I've included this example to show that even under favourable circumstances, it's rare to include 200 papers in a psychology meta-analysis. However, as time passes and more literature is published, the number of papers available for inclusion in a meta-analysis will increase. For now, you are unlikely to end up meta-analysing more than 50 studies, and most likely, may end up meta-analysing fewer than 20. As a result, a search that generates fewer, relevant, papers, seems to me the best way to proceed.

Having covered essential information about the first three steps of a systematic review, I'm going to end this chapter by covering PROSPERO—an online register of pre-registered protocols—and introducing PRISMA— guidelines for reporting results of a meta-analysis—as complementary methods to help make your meta-analysis replicable and transparent. I'll return to PRISMA when discussing how to write up the results of your meta in Chap. 15.

PROSPERO

PROSPERO is an online register maintained by the Centre for Systematic Reviews at the University of York, https://www.crd.york.ac.uk/PROSPERO/, and a key part of the systematic review process. PROSPERO encourages transparency of reporting by asking researchers to pre-register their systematic review with a view to reducing bias in reporting; by pre-registering your review, you are telling the world what you intend to do in your review before you do it. Pre-registration makes it harder to cherry pick findings at a later stage which can be an issue with systematic reviews, with reviewers tempted to present results in a particularly favourable light to avoid the perils of publication bias (see Chap. 13). Since its inception, PROSPERO has become one of the two main registers of secondary analyses, along with the Cochrane Library. Before you start any meta-analysis, I recommend you search both databases for existing reviews on your topic of interest. If a meta-analysis already exists on your topic, or a closely related topic, you might want to rethink your review area.

I first used PROSPERO to pre-register Cooke et al. (2023) and found it to be a simple process: you complete an online form, outlining your review questions, review team, inclusion criteria, et cetera. It is set up for traditional systematic reviews of RCTs, and maps onto PICO, but it is fairly easy to navigate. For meta-analyses, the PROSPERO team are keen on you providing precise information on how you plan to meta-analyse your data: What is your effect size? What method of pooling do you plan to use? How will you report heterogeneity? How will you identify publication bias? I will cover all these issues in detail in Chap. 7, when we cover data synthesis.

Three more things to say about PROSPERO. First, registration is an active process. The PROSPERO team will ask you to make changes to your submission if they do not feel it is sufficiently clear. While this can be frustrating it usually yields a better protocol. Second, when writing up your findings for submission to a journal, go back to your protocol for handy information, like What was your review question??! Or your inclusion criteria? The process of screening papers, data extraction, quality appraisal, and data synthesis takes time, so, it is worth going back to your protocol to remind yourself what the plan was at the start, as in my experience, it is all too easy to get side-tracked from what you originally proposed. Also, include your PROSPERO registration number in your publication as this is required by many journals. You may have to blind this information if you submit your meta to a journal that uses blind peer review, otherwise, a reviewer could look up who did the review! Finally, when you have finished your review, go back to PROSPERO and update the status of your review. This can seem daunting—admitting you are nearly finished with your review means losing some control over it—but it is essential to provide this update because it keeps the register current. PROSPERO contains 'ghost' registrations, for reviews that have been started but not published—don't add to their number. It is really satisfying to update your registration to published, so, don't forget to do this either. I recommend all meta-analyses are pre-registered as this increases the transparency of reviews.

PRISMA

PROSPERO is something to engage with at the start of your meta-analysis. I find it helps codify my thoughts on the meta-analysis I am about to do and provide a roadmap for screening, data extraction, quality appraisal, and data synthesis. In contrast, the Preferred Reporting of Information in Systematic Reviews and Meta-Analyses (PRISMA; Liberati et al., 2009) https://www.prisma-statement.org/, is something I tend to engage with following completion of screening. At this point, I complete the PRISMA flowchart detailed screening and identification of papers for inclusion in the meta-analysis. Just before I submit my meta-analysis I complete the PRISMA checklist to ensure I have included all the relevant information in my paper. Many journals insist on meta-analyses being reported in line with PRISMA.

Once you have decided on your final set of studies you can complete your PRISMA flowchart, which can be downloaded from the PRISMA website, because you know how many studies have been found in your searches and how many you have included/excluded at each step of screening. The flowchart illustrates this information in a really clear way.

The second part of the PRISMA process is to complete the PRISMA checklist, which is done right before submission of the paper to a journal. You do this last because the checklist asks you to specify on which page numbers you have reported various aspects of your meta-analysis. Doing this at the end means you know which page(s) in the final version of the paper contain these pieces of information. It won't take you more than 30 minutes to complete the checklist. We'll talk more about completing PRISMA processes when discussing writing up meta-analysis later in Chap. 15.

Summary

In this chapter, I have covered the essentials of the first three steps of conducting a systematic review as part of completing a meta-analysis. I have used some of my past review questions, inclusion/exclusion criteria and search terms and sources to show how I have completed systematic reviews as part of my meta-analyses, and I hope that offering these examples will help you complete the searching and screening part of your own systematic review prior to completing your meta-analysis. The next chapter will cover data extraction when conducting a meta-analysis.

References

Ajzen, I. (1991). The theory of planned behavior. *Organizational Behavior and Human Decision Processes, 50*, 179–211. https://doi.org/10.1016/0749-5978(91)90020-T

Ajzen, I., & Fishbein, M. (1973). Attitudinal and normative variables as predictors of specific behaviors. *Journal of Personality and Social Psychology, 27*, 41–57.

Birdi, G., Cooke, R., & Knibb, R. C. (2020). Impact of atopic dermatitis on quality of life in adults: A systematic review and meta-analysis. *International Journal of Dermatology, 59*(4). https://doi.org/10.1111/ijd.14763

Boland, A., Cherry, G., & Dickson, R. (2017). *Doing a systematic review: A student's guide* (2nd ed.). SAGE Publications.

Cooke, R., Dahdah, M., Norman, P., & French, D. P. (2016). How well does the theory of planned behaviour predict alcohol consumption? A systematic review and meta-analysis. *Health Psychology Review, 10*, 148–167. https://doi.org/10.1080/17437199.2014.947547

Cooke, R., & French, D. P. (2008). How well do the theory of reasoned action and theory of planned behaviour predict intentions and attendance at screening programmes? A meta-analysis. *Psychology & Health, 23*(7), 745–765. https://doi.org/10.1080/08870440701544437

Cooke, R., McEwan, H., & Norman, P. (2023). The effect of forming implementation intentions on alcohol consumption: A systematic review and meta-analysis. *Drug and Alcohol Review, 42*, 68–80. https://doi.org/10.1111/dar.13553

Cooke, R., & Sheeran, P. (2004). Moderation of cognition-intention and cognition-behaviour relations: A meta-analysis of properties of variables from the theory of planned behaviour. *The British Journal of Social Psychology, 43*(Pt 2), 159–186. https://doi.org/10.1348/0144666041501688

Hagger, M. S., Koch, S., Chatzisarantis, N. L. D., & Orbell, S. (2017). The common sense model of self-regulation: Meta-analysis and test of a process model. *Psychological Bulletin, 143*(11), 1117–1154. https://doi.org/10.1037/bul0000118

Hagger, M. S., & Orbell, S. (2003). A meta-analytic review of the common-sense model of illness representations. *Psychology & Health, 18*(2), 141–184. https://doi.org/10.1080/088704403100081321

Liberati, A., Altman, D. G., Tetzlaff, J., Mulrow, C., Gøtzsche, P. C., Ioannidis, J. P. A., Clarke, M., Devereaux, P. J., Kleijnen, J., & Moher, D. (2009). The PRISMA statement for reporting systematic reviews and meta-analyses of studies that evaluate health care interventions: Explanation and elaboration. *Journal of Clinical Epidemiology, 62*, e1–e34. https://doi.org/10.1016/j.jclinepi.2009.06.006

Newby, K., Teah, G., Cooke, R., Li, X., Brown, K., Salisbury-Finch, B., Kwah, K., Bartle, N., Curtis, K., Fulton, E., Parsons, J., Dusseldorp, E., & Williams, S. L. (2021). Do automated digital health behaviour change interventions have a positive effect on self-efficacy? A systematic review and meta-analysis. *Health Psychology Review, 15*(1), 140–158. https://doi.org/10.1080/17437199.2019.1705873

Todd, J., Kothe, E., Mullan, B., & Monds, L. (2016). Reasoned versus reactive prediction of behaviour: A meta-analysis of the prototype willingness model. *Health Psychology Review, 10*(1), 1–24. https://doi.org/10.1080/17437199.2014.922895

van Lettow, B., de Vries, H., Burdorf, A., & van Empelen, P. (2016). Quantifying the strength of the associations of prototype perceptions with behaviour, behavioural willingness and intentions: A meta-analysis. *Health Psychology Review, 10*(1), 25–43. https://doi.org/10.1080/17437199.2014.941997

Data Extraction for Meta-Analysis

5

Data Extraction for Meta-Analysis

A key difference between meta-analysis and systematic review is that when conducting a meta you are particularly interested in the statistical information reported by studies because, if a study does not report statistical information, it cannot easily be included in a meta-analysis. This difference between meta-analysis and systematic review has an important impact on how you think about applying your inclusion criteria during data extraction. In a systematic review, you typically specify an outcome of interest—blood pressure, physical activity, condom use, educational performance. As long as this outcome is measured in some way, you can often include the study in your systematic review, assuming other inclusion criteria are also met. In contrast, in a meta-analysis, your focus shifts from the outcome being present in some form in the paper to being used as part of a statistical test, that is, the outcome being correlated with a predictor of interest, or the outcome being compared between two groups at follow-up, or the same group over time. This shift in focus means that when you full-text screen papers for a meta-analysis, you must be able to extract statistical information to enable you to pool effect sizes in a meta-analysis. Failure to report statistical information is a valid reason for excluding a paper from a meta-analysis.

Before You Begin Data Extraction

Imagine that you have completed your systematic review and identified papers to include in your meta-analysis, that is, you've completed the first three steps of a systematic review as outlined in Chap. 4. The next step is to create a study characteristics table with the author names and years for the included studies in the

R. Cooke, *Meta-Analysis for Psychologists*,
https://doi.org/10.1007/978-3-031-73773-2_5

leftmost column and additional (blank) columns for the information you will extract. I also recommend you create a data extraction form at this stage to help consistently extract information from the included studies as discussed in the next section.

How to Get Started with Data Extraction When Conducting a Meta-Analysis

I would start by creating a data extraction form that contains fields for key information. In almost all forms, there are common fields: authors and year of publication, country of study, sample details. Inclusion of other fields depends on the study design and effect size. For instance, in a meta-analysis of effect size differences, you need to extract study design information, including the design (RCT, quasi-experiment, pre-post), follow-up time frame as well as information about the experimental manipulation/intervention content. I also like to code information about the content of the control condition as such information can often help you interpret the results of your meta-analysis. For the meta-analysis, you'll need to extract either (1) the means and standard deviations for the outcome(s), plus the sample sizes, for both the experimental/intervention and control/comparison groups or (2) the effect size and a measure of variance (sample error or study variance), if the authors have reported these. Either set of statistics is required to conduct the meta-analysis (see Chaps. 7 and 8). Alternatively, a form for a meta-analysis of correlations needs to extract the overall (total) sample size and extract at least one, and often, multiple correlations; in Cooke et al. (2016), we reported tests of eight theoretical relationships based on independent correlations. In the next two sections, I am going to show you how I extracted data from one study included in a correlational meta-analysis (Cooke et al., 2016), and separately, how I extracted data from one study included in an experimental meta-analysis (Cooke et al., 2023). I'll use the templates available on my Open Science Framework website https://osf.io/4zs5k.

Data Extraction for a Correlational Meta-Analysis

Table 5.1 shows you the completed data form for Paul Norman and Mark Conner's (2006) paper which was included in Cooke et al.'s (2016) meta-analysis of TPB alcohol studies.

Extracting study author names and year of study is an easy place to start—they are listed on the first page of the paper! It's sometimes harder to determine the country of study—it's amazing how many papers do not report this information in the methods section, with this paper being no exception. I think the main reason for this is to ensure that the study is blinded for peer review. In this case, I assumed that as both authors are affiliated with English universities, the study was conducted in England. When doing data extraction for meta-analyses, you often must make educated guesses like this. The rest of information you need to extract is reported in the methods and results sections of the paper. My tendency is to look for the

Table 5.1 Data extraction form for meta-analysis of correlations

Study label (authors + publication year)	Norman and Conner (2006)
Study location (country where data was collected)	England
Sample characteristics and recruitment	Undergraduate psychology students (mean age = 20.26, SD = 4.37; 92 male; 305 female, 1 missing). Not stated where recruitment took place.
Follow-up (s)	One week
Sample size(s)	Baseline $N = 398$; follow-up $N = 273$
Outcome(s)	(1) Binge drinking defined as: at least 5 pints of beer, or 10 shots or small glasses of wine for men; at least 3 and ½ pints of beer, 7 shots or small glasses of wine for women (2) Intentions
Correlates of outcome (1)	Intentions, perceived control, self-efficacy
Intention-binge drinking correlation	0.48
Perceived control-binge drinking correlation	−0.12
Self-efficacy-binge drinking correlation	0.42
Correlates of outcome (2)	Attitudes, subjective norms, perceived control, self-efficacy
Attitude-intention correlation	0.83
Subjective norm-intention correlation	0.43
Perceived control-intention correlation	−0.22
Self-efficacy-intention correlation	0.70

correlations which are often displayed in a correlation matrix, immediately after completing the Study Label and Study Location fields, because these values are the most important information for your meta-analysis. No correlations = no meta-analysis! In addition, most correlation studies are conducted using less complex study designs than experiments or interventions, which usually have intervention content, control group information, randomisation processes, et cetera to extract.

As is common in papers testing theoretical predictions, Paul and Mark included a correlation matrix that allowed me to quickly extract seven correlations from this paper, each representing theoretical relationships: attitude–intention; subjective norm–intention; perceived control–intention; self-efficacy–intention; intention–behaviour; perceived control–behaviour; self-efficacy–behaviour. When you write up your results, you should include these correlations in your table of study characteristics. They will also be entered into your meta-analysis for pooling. The other critical statistical information you need for your meta-analysis of correlations is the sample size each correlation is based on. As we shall see in Chap. 8, a meta-analysis of correlations involves three pieces of information: study label; sample size;

correlation—that's it!!! So, make sure you extract the sample sizes being mindful that sometimes sample sizes vary between relationships—check your paper carefully, especially notes below the correlation matrix.

After extracting correlations for the theoretical relationships—literally the most important information in this meta-analysis—I finished off the form by extracting information about the sample type (Undergraduate psychology students), sample demographics reported by authors (mean age (and standard deviation) or age range, number of male and female participants) and made a note about recruitment method. Some psychology papers talk about recruitment but not all do so; you may have to leave this blank. I also extracted the follow-up period which is important because this meta-analysis was looking at studies using prospective designs, that is, where behaviour is measured at a later time point to psychological predictors. There's a nice paper by Hagger and Hamilton (2023) on this issue that I recommend you read if you want to know more about such designs. My PhD was focused on the stability of cognitions, such as attitudes and intentions, over time, so I have usually looked at the time frame between measurement of constructs or behaviour and you may end up using this as a moderator variable (see Chap. 12).

Data Extraction for an Experimental Meta-Analysis

Table 5.2 shows the completed data extraction form from Chris Armitage's (2009) paper, which was included in Cooke et al. (2023). Like the correlational example, the first field contains the Study Authors and Publication Year. Chris also reports the study location in the method section (North of England) and information on the sample representativeness, which is quite rare in psychology papers. The fourth field—Intervention description—is really important when doing data extraction for a meta-analysis of effect size differences. Include as much information as you need here as this is a field you are likely to use when interpreting the results of your meta-analysis.

The fifth field—Control description—is also important in my opinion. Sometimes what the control groups did (or did not do) can impact on interpretation of the results of your meta-analysis (see De Bruin et al., 2021; Kraiss et al., 2023, for more).

The next three fields are quite specific to this meta-analysis and may not be needed in your meta-analysis. First, in many papers in this literature, researchers combined implementation intention interventions with other interventions, usually focused on increasing motivation, so, it was useful to code if the intervention was a stand-alone or part of a combined intervention. Coding this information allowed us to run an exploratory analysis to see if receiving the intervention in combination or as a stand-alone intervention affected effect size differences, which it did not. Second, when we pre-registered our protocol on PROSPERO, we thought that mode of delivery (i.e. face-to-face, online, paper) and follow-up time point(s) might both moderate the overall effect size. So, we recorded information about these factors on our form. I'll talk more about moderators in Chap. 12.

Table 5.2 Data extraction form for meta-analysis of effect size differences

Study label (authors + publication year)	Armitage (2009)
Study location (country where data was collected)	England
Sample characteristics and recruitment	Shopping malls and working environments; 18–74 years old (M = 38.4; SD = 15.46) 125/113 women (53%) to men; 92% white (educational qualifications also noted)
Intervention description	If-then plans: Self-generated implementation intention; experimenter generated implementation intention
Control description	Two control conditions: Passive control: mere measurement Active control: asked to plan how to reduce their alcohol consumption but not provided with any guidance on how to do this
Standalone/combined	Stand-alone
Mode of delivery	Face-to-face
Follow-up timepoint(s)	One month
Outcome(s)	Weekly drinking
Control sample size	24* (passive control); 21 (active control)
Intervention sample size	18* (self-generated implementation intention); 16 (experimenter-generated implementation intention)
Statistics reported in paper	Means + SDs
Control mean/SD for BD	5.49 (2.94)
Intervention mean/SD for BD	4.42 (2.70)

Notes:

- Samples were split into low- and high-risk groups based on past drinking. Effect sizes were only calculated for the high-risk groups as there was no effect of the intervention in low-risk groups
- We decided to compute the effect size difference between the self-generated implementation intention and passive control because this is the comparison done in most other included studies

Finally, the outcome(s) field is essential in meta-analyses of effect size differences. To meet our inclusion criteria, studies had to report measuring weekly alcohol consumption and/or heavy episodic drinking (binge drinking). In this case, weekly alcohol consumption was the outcome reported and so was recorded on the form. Coding for the correct outcome, when there are multiple potential outcomes, which helps to ensure that the data is included in the correct meta-analysis.

Following the outcome(s) field, we have the raw materials of a meta-analysis of effect size differences: the sample sizes, means, and standard deviations for both experimental (intervention) and control (comparison) groups. With these six pieces of information, plus a study label, you can perform an experimental meta-analysis (see Chap. 10). If you have more than one outcome, you are advised to add rows to the bottom of the form to capture the statistics for each effect size.

Hopefully, these completed forms give you an idea of the information you need to extract for your meta-analysis. To summarise, some information needs to be extracted in all meta-analyses (Authors and Year, Study Country, Sample Characteristics). Other information depends on the type of meta-analysis you are doing, for example, correlations for a meta-analysis of correlations, means, standard deviations, sample sizes for intervention and control groups or effect sizes and a measure of variance for a meta-analysis of effect size differences). Sample size in a meta-analysis of correlations is typically the total sample. Sample sizes in meta-analysis of effect size differences reflect samples in each group. Additional information, driven by the focus of your meta, including moderators and information about the study you need, can be added to your extraction forms which should be made bespoke to your meta-analysis. Feel free to adapt these forms available on the Open Science Framework (https://osf.io/4zs5k) or create your own.

A Note on Data Extraction Forms That Already Exist

As there are already data extraction forms you can download and use, you might wonder why I have not recommended using them? It's mainly because I'm familiar with my forms, and that because I created them they fit my needs. That's not to say available forms are bad or should not be used. If you find a form you like, then use it. Alternatively, use my forms. Or create your own. What really matters is that you are consistent in how you extract data, across studies, and I'm not sure there is any form that will do that for you!

The Advantages of Independent Data Extraction

When I started conducting meta-analyses in 1999, it never occurred to me to get someone to check my data extraction; the information is all there in the paper—how difficult could it be to extract it? While I still think data extraction is straightforward, I now routinely ask another reviewer to independently complete data extraction. For example, I asked Mary Dahdah, an ex-MSc Health Psychology student from when I worked at Aston University to do this for Cooke et al. (2016). It's a good quality assurance practice to get into the habit of doing. Chances are, your reviewer buddy will extract exactly the same data as you, but maybe there are some discrepancies that make it worth doing. You sometimes find papers that report multiple sample sizes, for instance, and extracting the right one, that is, the one that the statistics are based on, can be challenging. Getting someone to check your extraction is well worth the effort. We recommend to our Professional Doctorate in Health Psychology Students that they get their independent rater to check at least 10% of the included studies. At the end of the process, we ask them to calculate a Kappa statistic to indicate the extent of inter-rater reliability.

What to Do When the Statistical Information You Want Has Not Been Reported?

The final section of this chapter focuses on what happens when the information you are looking to extract is not reported in the paper, or online; sometimes researchers upload information that they cannot fit into the word count of the paper onto the Open Science Framework. Assuming the information you want is not available, what are your options?

The simplest option is to contact the authors and request the information you need. I have had several lovely email exchanges with authors about data from their research—I get the feeling that they rarely hear from the wider world about their work and are happy when they receive emails requesting information. I've had researchers post me chapters of their PhD (hard copy, air mailed!), dig out old data from long-completed studies and send me SPSS data files of additional analyses. I always thank them for their efforts by email and make sure I note this generous activity in the published meta-analysis in the acknowledgments section (see Chap. 15). I also see it as a point of principle that if I am asked for information I always try and provide it. Reciprocity makes the world a better place. I would argue that the action of contacting authors to request data does not necessarily undermine the systematic nature of your meta-analysis, although, if not all authors respond to your request, you do run the risk of potentially biasing the result of your meta-analysis via a form of reporting bias (see Chap. 6). This form of reporting bias is bias in the statistical information you have available to pool due to decisions made by authors about what they report in the paper. There's not too much you can do about this, but you should be aware of it as a potential issue if not all authors you contact respond.

Ultimately, you can exclude papers that do not report the statistics you need, although I believe this drastic move requires some justification. One scenario that would justify such an approach is when you are under time pressure to complete your meta-analysis and do not have time to wait to hear from authors. Further justification for exclusion is, in my experience, you only end up with a few studies that do not report the information you require. So, you could argue that excluding the papers that do not report statistics is unlikely to affect the pooled effect sizes generated during meta-analyses too much. That is quite a judgment call to make, and I would rather try to get the information from authors, although I do acknowledge that this approach won't work every time. Another option is to convert information that is reported into an effect size you can use, for example, in Cooke and Sheeran (2004), we calculated a phi coefficient, a correlation based on frequency data, to enable us to retain a paper within our analysis. Borentstein et al. (2021) Chap. 7 has further information on how to convert effect sizes.

Summary

The aim of this chapter was to get you thinking about data extraction for meta-analyses by providing examples of completed data extraction forms for you to see how I conducted data extraction. I'll end with a couple of top tips for data extraction.

Top tips for data extraction:

- Read and re-read your papers multiple times to check you have the correct statistical and methodological information.
- Ask a review buddy to data extract at least 10% of included studies to check you agree on information (especially things like sample sizes, correlations, and descriptive statistics). It's essential to extract the correct statistical information as making errors means redoing the meta-analyses.
- Keep a folder of data extraction forms for easy access to information when you are interpreting results of your meta-analysis (especially moderator analyses).

Tasks

Practise Data Extraction by completing these two tasks:

Task 1: Complete data extraction using the blank form for Norman's (2011) paper (see reference list) for inclusion in a meta-analysis of correlations.

Task 2: Complete data extraction using the blank form for Hagger et al.'s (2012) paper (see reference list) for inclusion in a meta-analysis of effect size differences.

References

Armitage, C. J. (2009). Effectiveness of experimenter-provided and self-generated implementation intentions to reduce alcohol consumption in a sample of the general population: A randomized exploratory trial. *Health Psychology, 28*, 545–553. https://doi.org/10.1037/a0015984

Cooke, R., Dahdah, M., Norman, P., & French, D. P. (2016). How well does the theory of planned behaviour predict alcohol consumption? A systematic review and meta-analysis. *Health Psychology Review, 10*, 148–167. https://doi.org/10.1080/17437199.2014.947547

Cooke, R., McEwan, H., & Norman, P. (2023). The effect of forming implementation intentions on alcohol consumption: A systematic review and meta-analysis. *Drug and Alcohol Review, 42*, 68–80. https://doi.org/10.1111/dar.13553

Cooke, R., & Sheeran, P. (2004). Moderation of cognition-intention and cognition-behaviour relations: A meta-analysis of properties of variables from the theory of planned behaviour. *The British Journal of Social Psychology, 43*(Pt 2), 159–186. https://doi.org/10.1348/0144666041501688

De Bruin, M., Black, N., Javornik, N., Viechtbauer, W., Eisma, M. C., Hartman-Boyce, J., Williams, A. J., West, R., Michie, S., & Johnston, M. (2021). Underreporting of the active content of behavioural interventions: A systematic review and meta-analysis of randomised trials of smoking cessation interventions. *Health Psychology Review, 15*(2), 195–213. https://doi.org/10.1080/17437199.2019.1709098

Hagger, M. S., & Hamilton, K. (2023). Longitudinal tests of the theory of planned behaviour: A meta-analysis. *European Review of Social Psychology, 1–57*. https://doi.org/10.1080/10463283.2023.2225897

Hagger, M. S., Lonsdale, A., Koka, A., Hein, V., Pasi, H., Lintunen, T., & Chatzisarantis, N. L. D. (2012). An intervention to reduce alcohol consumption in undergraduate students using implementation intentions and mental simulations: A cross-national study. *International Journal of Behavioral Medicine, 19*, 82–96. https://doi.org/10.1007/s12529-011-9163-8

Kraiss, J., Viechtbauer, W., Black, N., Johnston, M., Hartmann-Boyce, J., Eisma, M., Javornik, N., Bricca, A., Michie, S., West, R., & De Bruin, M. (2023). Estimating the true effectiveness of smoking cessation interventions under variable comparator conditions: A systematic review and meta-regression. *Addiction, 118*(10), 1835–1850. https://doi.org/10.1111/add.16222

Norman, P. (2011). The theory of planned behavior and binge drinking among undergraduate students: Assessing the impact of habit strength. *Addictive Behaviors, 36*(5), 502–507. https://doi.org/10.1016/j.addbeh.2011.01.025

Norman, P., & Conner, M. (2006). The theory of planned behaviour and binge drinking: Assessing the moderating role of past behaviour within the theory of planned behaviour. *British Journal of Health Psychology, 11*(Pt 1), 55–70. https://doi.org/10.1348/135910705X43741

Quality Appraisal for Meta-Analysis

6

What Is Quality Appraisal?

Quality appraisal is the process used to assess the quality of research studies included in a systematic review. High quality studies use stronger research designs that reduce the likelihood of biases influencing interpretation of results (see Fig. 6.1). For example, if you randomly allocate participants to condition, your study is of higher quality than a similar study that does not do so because randomisation ensures that factors which may affect performance in each condition, like participants' motivation to change their behaviour, the extent of their impairment, or the time they take to engage with the intervention, are less likely to influence scores on the outcome. Randomisation addresses selection bias, which is one of several biases we assess when we quality appraise studies included in our meta-analysis.

This chapter will begin by introducing biases assessed in quality appraisal to prime you to understand the tools we use for quality appraisal, which are mainly focused on identifying the presence or absence of various biases. After describing each bias, I have included text to outline methods researchers can use to address biases; by telling you what methods researchers use to address biases, you'll find it easier to spot them in your included studies when conducting quality appraisal for your meta-analysis. I have taken the decision to begin by focusing on experimental study designs because the principles of quality appraisal for experimental studies are more clearly developed than equivalent principles for correlational study designs, which have only recently received attention.

R. Cooke, *Meta-Analysis for Psychologists*,
https://doi.org/10.1007/978-3-031-73773-2_6

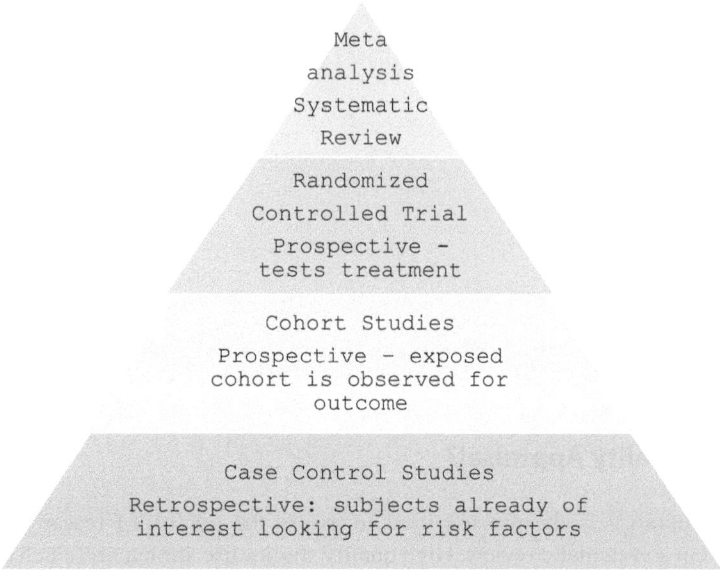

Fig. 6.1 Evidence pyramid

Biases in Research Studies

I'm going to introduce you to five biases—Selection bias; Performance Bias; Detection Bias; Attrition Bias; and Reporting Bias—that form the basis of the Cochrane Risk of Bias tool (Higgins & Green, 2011), which is commonly used to quality appraise studies. I'll begin with Selection Bias as this is the first row of the form.

Selection Bias (Part 1)

When conducting a study using an experimental design, it is important that you control for individual differences between groups. If there are differences between the two groups, these differences could explain why you found an effect rather than your experiment or intervention. It is common practice to run inferential tests to determine if the groups differ on baseline measures such as the outcome, predictor variables, or demographic factors. If tests show no difference between the groups on these variables, researchers often take this as a good sign because null results indicate that the two groups are similar at baseline, that is, before participants receive the experimental manipulation or intervention materials. Groups being similar at baseline makes it more justifiable to claim that differences in an outcome at follow-up are due to receiving or not receiving the intervention.

However, because it is impossible to measure **all** the variables that might differ between groups in any study, such tests offer only indirect support for the claim that the groups do not differ at baseline; they do not differ on variables you measured, but they may differ on variables you didn't! Let us say you **do not** measure how motivated people are to change their behaviour. If you have **not** randomly allocated participants to condition then you could end up accidentally assigning all the people who are really motivated to change their behaviour to receive the intervention, and everyone who aren't really motivated end up in the control group. You may well find that your intervention 'successfully' changes your outcome in the desired direction at follow-up. You may well attribute this outcome to your brilliant intervention, when the reality is that you were lucky that the more motivated participants all received the intervention, and the less motivated participants received the control materials. If allocation had been the other way round, perhaps the results would not have been so impressive.

Random allocation to group neatly solves this issue. You may still be unaware of participants' motivation, but random allocation to condition will almost certainly spread the more motivated participants to the intervention and control groups evenly, making it more likely that a 'successful' intervention result, that is, a change in an outcome at follow-up, is due to the brilliance of your intervention rather than factors that differ between the groups. Randomising participants with an almost even chance of receiving the intervention or experimental manipulation vs the control condition, with a large enough sample, protects against selection bias. Random allocation drastically reduces the odds of individual differences affecting your interpretation of the effect of your intervention or manipulation. It's all about minimising the probability that something happens.

Methods Researchers Use to Randomly Allocate Participants to Condition

In the past, researchers used random number tables, or random telephone dialling methods, to randomly allocate participants to condition. Nowadays, researchers tend to use websites that generate random number sequences such as www.random.org, or the brilliantly named The Sealed Envelope, or randomisation functions within survey software—Qualtrics can randomly allocate participants to condition.

Selection Bias (Part 2)

When I first started using the Cochrane Risk of Bias tool to quality appraise studies, it took me some time to get my head around the difference between allocation concealment and blinding of participants and personnel (see Performance Bias section); how is allocation concealment different to blinding? In brief, allocation concealment relates to selection bias—who ends up in which condition—whereas blinding is about performance bias—how participants and personnel act if they know which group they are in. Allocation concealment and blinding are related processes that address different biases. The point of judging allocation concealment is to provide a complementary perspective on selection bias. Just because you randomise participants to condition does not mean you are protecting yourself against all forms of selection bias. If you know what condition you are in, or, if the team running the study know what condition you are in, it has the potential to introduce bias. As a lapsed social psychologist, I do like a bit of deception in my studies, so, by nature I tend to conceal allocation to condition. What I don't always do is report this in the papers I write, which can make it hard to judge the risk of bias for allocation concealment.

Methods Researchers Use to Conceal Allocation to Condition from Participants

One of the best ways to conceal allocation to condition from participants is to have someone outside of the research team allocate participants to groups. In Randomized Controlled Trials (RCTs), this is usually done by a member of the clinical trials unit, who are responsible for running the trial, but not part of the main project team. This provides an extra layer of secrecy to the project to help reduce selection bias. Many psychology studies are not RCTs, however, and as a result, the researchers may have limited resources to employ someone to independently allocate participants to condition. In this case, researchers can use computer software to allocate to condition. Programmes like Gorilla and survey packages like Qualtrics contain functions for random allocation to condition. Using these methods helps reduce selection bias.

Performance Bias

Psychologists are taught a lot about performance bias as part of their training in experimental research methodology as undergraduates; as a discipline we are acutely aware that if participants know they are in the experimental/intervention group this can affect their performance. They might try harder to complete a puzzle or pay more attention when receiving an intervention. Alternatively, knowing you are in the control group can lead to reduced persistence on a task or disinterest when completing measures. Psychologists are also aware that researchers may intentionally or unintentionally influence participants' performance. Overall, I would say that psychologists are aware of the importance of blinding participants to group and aware that blinding personnel, where practical, can be a good idea too. In sum, failing to blind participants and personnel to group allocation can introduce performance bias.

Methods Researchers Use to Blind Participants and Personnel to Condition

Psychologists generally have a good understanding of ways in which you can blind participants to condition, which include options such as (1) using a sealed envelope to conceal from researchers and students which group participants are in or (2) minimal differences in manipulation instructions between control and experimental groups.

For example, in Cooke et al. (2014), we used both methods: the control group read text that contained the word least, whereas the experimental group read text that contained the word most—that was the only difference between groups! We handed materials over using sealed envelopes (see Box 6.1) based on a random sequence, meaning we were addressing selection bias as well as performance bias.

> **Box 6.1 Counteracting Selection and Performance Bias** In Cooke et al. (2014), we wanted to see if asking one group of participants to self-affirm, by focusing on a valued aspect of their self-concept like honesty or reliability prior to reading a health message about the benefits of being active, would lead them to increase their activity levels compared with a group not asked to self-affirm. I decided to use a double-blind procedure to increase the chance that effects we found were not due to performance bias. Prior to data collection taking place, I generated a random sequence for allocation to the two groups using www.random.org. I then printed out study materials and filled envelopes for the two groups, creating one pile of control group envelopes and one of experimental group envelopes. Finally, I ordered the envelopes using the random sequence and handed them to the researcher conducting data collection. They, nor the participants, knew which condition they were in, and because I was not collecting data myself, I was satisfied that performance bias was unlikely to be an issue in this study.

Detection Bias

To understand detection bias, it is instructive to think about how statistical analyses are conducted in other disciplines. In medicine, statisticians run analyses of RCTs. This has one major advantage when thinking about risk of bias; the statisticians are merely doing their job, by running statistical tests. Their stake in the results of a study—the desire to show that an intervention is 'successful'—is minimal. When the analyses are finished, they write them up and then move on to working on the next trial. It's hard to see how they would be tempted to bias results by, for example, excluding cases that do not fit the desired pattern. The process of having an independent party conduct the analyses is called blinding of outcome assessors; the statisticians are literally assessing the outcome, using statistics.

This approach contrasts sharply with the way things are done in psychology. Most psychologists conducting quantitative studies run their own analyses so, undergraduate and postgraduate psychology students are trained to run their own analyses and develop skills and confidence in doing so. Developing statistical skills is a core part of all UK psychology programmes accredited by the British Psychological Society and most UK psychology postgraduate programmes, including being a core element of MSc Health Psychology programmes I've taught on.

Because psychologists run their own statistical analyses it typically means they have unblinded access to the data, indicating which participants are in which groups, when running statistical tests. This opens the door to detection bias and p-hacking (see Box 6.2).

The major giveaway that psychologists have a blind spot about detection bias is the rarity with which blinding of outcome assessors is mentioned in psychology studies. Indeed, it was only when I completed quality appraisal for Cooke et al. (2023) that I thought about it at all and noticed that all of my included studies were rated as high risk of bias for detection bias. Because psychologists analyse their own data or get their students/researchers to do it for them, we need to be aware of detection bias.

Box 6.2 Imaginary Example of Detection Bias Imagine you want to compare the effect of your intervention on physical activity between the control and intervention groups, so you run an independent groups t-test. Your output shows you that the direction of the effect is as you expected; participants who received the intervention increased their physical activity while participants in the control group maintained their activity levels. However, the magnitude of the effect size is small ($d = 0.21$) and the test fails to meet conventional levels of significance, that is, $p = 0.06$. You know that a paper based on a significant result is more likely to be accepted for publication in a top journal (see Chap. 13). As you are the outcome assessor you might be tempted to engage in *p*-hacking—you go looking for 'outliers' in either your control or intervention group. Maybe you find that five of your control group increased their physical activity at follow-up and you find some grounds for treating them as outliers, for example, they were more physically active at baseline than other control group participants. Alternatively, maybe five of your intervention group participants maintained their physical activity at follow-up. Perhaps they missed some of the intervention sessions and it could be argued that they should not be included in the main analysis. Removing either set of five participants magically transforms the significance from $p = 0.06$ into $p = 0.04$, and although your effect size remains small ($d = 0.28$), you now have a significant effect of your intervention on your outcome, and publication in a top journal looks possible!

Showing an intervention worked is a major incentive to mess with the data. On Retraction Watch's website http://retractiondatabase.org/RetractionSearch.aspx? you will see several psychologists listed there, including Diederik Stapel, who made up his results for prestige and career advancement https://www.theguardian.com/science/2012/sep/13/scientific-research-fraud-bad-practice.

I believe the main way to overcome detection bias in psychology is for more psychological research to be funded. Much psychological research is completed without any funding, which is another key difference with other disciplines. Until psychologists conduct research studies with funds to employ an outcome assessor to provide an independent statistical evaluation of results, I believe that detection bias will remain an almost ever-present risk in psychological research. Even when you have money to employ an outcome assessor to run the analyses, there will likely be psychologists who *enjoy* analysing data—like me!—and will prefer to run their own analyses. Perhaps these individuals can be given the dataset after someone independently confirms the results, to reduce the risk of detection bias.

Methods Researchers Use to Blind Outcome Assessors

In medicine, statisticians are employed to run statistical analyses on RCTs, providing an outcome assessor who is blind to the study's research questions, thus protecting against detection bias. Don't be surprised if there is no mention of efforts to avoid detection bias in papers reporting psychology studies, although some research teams are large enough to replicate what is done in medicine by having an independent assessor of the outcomes who can be blinded to research questions.

Attrition Bias

Attrition bias occurs when there is a difference between the sample you recruit and the sample you analyse. For instance, imagine you recruit 100 students into a study about binge drinking, but are only able to retain 50 at follow-up—you have lost half of your sample between baseline and follow-up, which has the potential to cause attrition bias. In this case, you only have responses from 50% of the original sample, which will limit generalizability of findings because the 50% of your baseline sample may differ on variables you are interested in from the 50% of the sample you have lost.

In Radtke et al. (2017), we found that those who dropped out of our intervention study at follow-up drank more alcohol at baseline relative to those who we retained in the study, meaning our intervention evaluation was undermined because we did not know what happened to consumption in those we lost. Attrition bias can also occur when you have incomplete data, that is, how you handle attrition, either statistically, by inputting missing values, for example, or by how you choose to include/exclude cases in your analysis.

To calculate the attrition rate in your study (1) subtract the follow-up sample size from the baseline sample size [telling you how many participants you lost] then (2) divide that value by the baseline sample size, finally (3) multiply by 100, to get the proportion of the original sample you lost. Here are some numbers to show this effect in action:

- Baseline sample = 250
- Follow-up sample = 179

- Difference between samples = 71
- Attrition rate = (71/250) × 100 = 28.4%

In this example, the attrition rate was 28.4%. You can also work out your retention rate (how many people completed both measures) by subtracting the attrition rate from 100. The retention rate is 71.6%.

I don't recall too many conversations about what a good/bad/average/poor attrition or retention rate is, although I do recall having a paper rejected for having a retention rate of 48%. While I was cross about the rejection at the time, I now appreciate the editor was correct to challenge the attrition in that study. I think most psychologists rely on heuristics to satisfy their desire to get their work published, although, I have not systematically researched this issue.

Other disciplines are much stricter on attrition rates. When I first read the Cochrane Guidelines for Risk of Bias, I was surprised that they were recommending that an attrition rate of 5% was desirable and evidence of low risk of bias. 5%!!! Apart from some of my early studies, which students completed in return for research credit, I rarely achieve a 5% attrition rate. When you do lots of prospective, and longitudinal, studies, with student samples, you come to expect attrition, with participants dropping out of follow-up surveys for a variety of reasons. Reading the guidelines further, the implication was that while between 6 and 10% attrition could be considered unclear risk of bias, anything more than 10% was clear evidence of high risk of bias. In other words, unless you retained 90% of your original sample, your study was at high risk of attrition bias.

When we are told something that challenges our world view, or we don't like, our natural tendency is to try and undermine it, because reconciling the information with what we know and accept may not be possible. As we shall see when I talk about using the Cochrane Risk of Bias tool in the next section, when I applied the threshold of 10% attrition bias to the studies in Cooke et al. (2023), most did not meet it. Interestingly, most of the study authors did not comment on attrition being an issue; where it was, analyses were often run using statistical measures to deal with missing data, like multiple imputation or running intention to treat analyses.

The issue of what psychologists consider acceptable levels of attrition is not one that is widely discussed. I believe this issue needs addressing in research methodology training and would benefit from psychologists, as a discipline, getting together to talk about this issue. I think because much psychological research is unfunded that we should expect higher levels of attrition than are found in RCTs, which potentially set a high benchmark because participants may be more invested in taking part in a trial, for example, when it relates to a treatment for a health condition, than they would be for a typical psychology survey study. Perhaps a good first step would be for psychologists to routinely comment on the power of their study based on the analysed (final) dataset. Power calculations are becoming more common in primary papers, but these sometimes talk about power based on baseline rather than final sample sizes, which can be misleading.

Methods Researchers Use to Reduce Attrition

Researchers use various statistical methods to reduce attrition, including multiple imputations or running intention to treat analyses. You can also look for information about retention methods reported in the method section of included studies. For instance, were incentives offered to participants for completing each wave of the study?

Reporting Bias

Reporting bias is sometimes called selective reporting. In the Cochrane Risk of Bias tool, it mentions selective outcome reporting, which makes me think of examples where authors have switched outcome after running statistical analyses. Box 6.3 gives an example of what I mean.

> **Box 6.3 Switching Outcomes After Running Statistical Analyses** You are interested in testing how well a school-based intervention effects children's fruit and vegetable intake, attitudes towards fruit and vegetable, and knowledge of the 5-a-day message. Before the study, your focus is on evaluating the effect of the intervention on fruit and vegetable intake as you decide this is the most important variable to show a change in. You designate fruit and vegetable intake as your primary outcome and attitudes and knowledge as secondary outcomes. When you run the analysis, as is often the case, the intervention has not changed fruit and vegetable intake ($d = 0.00$). On the other hand, the intervention led to positive changes in attitudes ($d = 0.30$) and knowledge ($d = 0.75$). Despite knowing that it is typically easier to show an intervention can change knowledge or attitudes than intake, you decide to switch the focus of your paper to emphasise the changes in knowledge and attitudes and de-emphasise the lack of change in intake. Doing this is an example of reporting bias and HARKing—Hypothesising After the Results are Known (Chambers, 2017).

I believe that reporting bias is partly a function of publication bias; if journals, and their editors, were more willing to publish null or negative results, then there would be less pressure on authors to jazz up their findings, and even less incentive for researchers to switch from one outcome to another, searching for the magical $p < 0.05$ effect. Following the Open Science Movement, I hope there will be less issues with reporting bias. One of the best things about Open Science is that it forces the research team to specify their primary and secondary outcomes prior to conducting the study. Most RCTs now publish a protocol paper outlining these decisions, while other authors use Open Science Framework, or other websites such as

AsPredicted, to guard against outcome switching. Hopefully, as time passes, outcome switching will become less of an issue. Having covered various biases you look for in quality appraisal of experimental designs, in the next section I'm going to talk through how we quality appraised studies included in Cooke et al. (2023).

Quality Appraising Experimental Studies as Part of a Meta-Analysis

When pre-registering the review protocol on PROSPERO for what became Cooke et al. (2023), we opted to use the Cochrane Risk of Bias tool. This tool seemed a good fit for the studies we were appraising. My co-author Helen McEwan and I used it to independently judge the risk of bias in the included studies. The form we used has been updated and is available online https://sites.google.com/site/riskofbiastool/.

For readers unfamiliar with this tool, you judge each included study on seven criteria: Random sequence generation; Allocation concealment; Blinding of participants and personnel; Blinding of outcome assessment; Incomplete outcome data; Selective reporting; and Other bias. These criteria map onto the biases covered in the previous section.[1] For each criterion, you judge the study as being low, unclear, or high risk of bias. Low risk of bias suggests you think that the bias you are rating is unlikely. Unclear risk of bias suggests you are unsure about the extent of bias, based on how the study was reported. Finally, high risk of bias suggests that there is a good chance that the study suffered from this bias. Next, I will talk through how I used the form for one of the studies included in Cooke et al. (2023).

Example Risk of Bias Form—Wittleder et al. (2019)

I've included the completed worksheet for Wittleder et al.'s (2019) study as Table 6.1. I've selected this paper because it was simple to quality appraise in some ways but not others.

Selection Bias (Random Sequence Generation and Allocation Concealment)

Wittleder et al. reported using Qualtrics to randomise participants to condition. So, I judged the paper to be low risk for selection bias; it seemed to me that there was a low risk of selection bias because Qualtrics handled randomisation. I judged papers which stated that participants were randomised to condition, but failed to mention how this happened, as unclear risk of selection bias. Mentioning randomisation is in the study's favour, but a failure to report the method used means I cannot know if

[1] Other bias is a catch-all category for biases not covered in the rest of the form.

Table 6.1 Assessment of bias: Wittleder et al. (2019)

Criteria	High risk	Low risk	Unclear risk of bias[a]	Comments
Random sequence generation—Selection bias (biased allocation to interventions) due to inadequate generation of a randomised sequence.				
		X		Randomisation performed by Qualtrics. They don't mention blocks but do talk about even randomised via Qualtrics survey flow. It is highly likely that allocation was random.
Allocation concealment—Selection bias due to inadequate concealment of allocations prior to assignment.				
		X		Qualtrics allocated participants to condition so allocation was concealed from participants and researchers.
Blinding of participants and personnel—Performance bias due to knowledge of the allocation interventions by participants and personnel performing the study.				
		X		Qualtrics allocated participants to condition. Paper reports that participants were blind to condition. Likely that researchers were too.
Blinding of outcome assessment—Detection bias due to knowledge of the allocated interventions by the outcome assessors.				
	X			No report of blinding of outcomes assessors.
Incomplete outcome data—Attrition bias due to amount, nature or handling of incomplete data.				
	X			Forty-Five per cent attrition. Report analyses that there were no condition differences in attrition rate and completers did not differ from non-completers on study variables
Selective reporting—Reporting bias due to selective outcome reporting.				
		X		
Other bias—Bias due to problems not covered elsewhere in the table.				
		X		

Bias assessment template based on The Cochrane Collaboration's tool for assessing risk of bias
[a]NB: Word limits in publications may lead to gaps in reporting which makes a bias assessment unclear

selection bias occurred. I reserved high risk of bias rating for papers that do not report randomisation to condition. Authors conducting experiments/evaluating interventions should aim to limit possible explanations of their results. Randomisation is one way to do this, and is often under the control of the authors, so failure to randomise merits a high risk of bias rating.

I judged the risk of bias for allocation concealment to be low for Wittleder et al.'s paper. With Qualtrics randomising to condition, it seems unlikely that there was bias in allocation to condition. It's worth noting that the authors made no reference to allocation concealment, so I did have to infer this when judging the paper as low risk of bias. Helen McEwan, the second author of the paper who independently rated each paper using the same form, and I decided that studies using computer-administered allocation to condition are likely to be low risk of bias. We reserved unclear risk of bias for studies that did not clearly report their method of allocation. We did not judge any of included studies to be high risk of bias.

Performance Bias (Blinding of Participants and Personnel)

I judged the risk of performance bias to be low in Wittleder et al.'s study. With Qualtrics randomly allocating participants to condition it is hard to see how participants could know which condition they were in, and this judgment was reported by the authors too. I think that the authors were blind to condition until data analyses were conducted. Other papers were rated as unclear for blinding—this was generally where no information was provided about how participants were blinded to condition, but it was not immediately obvious that participants and researchers were aware of conditions. As noted above, I believe that psychologists are acutely aware of blinding, so it is perhaps not too surprising that we judged all the studies in our meta-analysis as low or unclear for performance bias.

Detection Bias (Blinding of Outcome Assessors)

In contrast to previous criteria, I rated Wittleder et al.'s study as high risk of detection bias. The authors made no mention of blinding outcome assessors, so, I had to assume that they ran analyses themselves. Indeed, we rated all the papers included in Cooke et al. (2023) as high risk of detection bias as none of them made any reference to blinding outcome assessors. When all papers in a meta-analysis suffer the same negative assessment, it is worth discussing the suitability of the tool for psychological research, which we did at the end of the paper. There is a broader point to be made about the suitability of tools designed for RCTs being used to evaluate experimental psychology studies. Although both study designs are experiments, the way research is reported is quite different. Perhaps psychologists should create their own tools.

Attrition Bias (Incomplete Outcome Data)

Wittleder et al. (2019) reported an attrition rate of 45%. As noted above, this eclipses the cut-off of 90% for unclear risk of bias and 95% for low risk of bias found in the Cochrane guidance. In the limitations section of the paper, the authors note that the attrition rate in their study was higher than typically found in clinical trials. There is not much the authors could do about this, beyond noting that attrition did not differ by condition, which is a positive finding. Most of the studies included in Cooke et al. (2023) reported high risk for attrition bias, although there were a couple of studies that reported zero or low levels of attrition indicating that it is possible for psychology papers to be rated as low risk of bias for incomplete outcome data.

Reporting Bias (Selective Reporting) and Other Bias (Bias Due to Problems Not Covered Elsewhere in the Table)

Helen and I judged that all included studies were low risk for both reporting bias and other bias. This is not to say either criterion won't be an issue with quality appraisal for your meta-analysis, just that it was not an issue for our studies. One final thing to note is that none of our included studies published a protocol paper outlining their plans prior to conducting the study. When you are quality appraising a literature where publication of protocols is accepted practice this makes the job of judging reporting bias potentially easier as you can compare the primary outcome mentioned in the protocol to the outcome reported in the paper. So, our quality appraisal is a qualified one on reporting bias; we did not find any evidence of it, but it was hard for us to do so due to the nature of the way the studies were conducted. The final section of this chapter will discuss quality appraisal of correlational studies.

Quality Appraising Correlational Studies

Because I am not as experienced at quality appraisal as the other steps of systematic reviewing, I found this a difficult chapter to write. This goes back to my training in meta-analyses of correlational studies. When I was trained to conduct meta-analysis, I did not spend a lot of time thinking about study quality. For my first meta-analysis (Cooke & Sheeran, 2004) there were not many papers available for inclusion so there was no way I could afford to be picky about which studies were included; if a study met the inclusion criteria, it was in, whether it was well conducted or not!

A key change in my thinking took place when I moved to Aston University and started to teach MSc Health Psychology students about systematic reviewing and meta-analysis. I discussed quality appraisal with my colleague Professor Helen Pattison, who had previously worked in a public health department at the University of Birmingham. Helen educated me on the differences between systematic reviews and meta-analysis, and particularly the importance of study quality, an issue I was blissfully unaware of! The quality of a trial is a big issue, with results having the potential to make a major impact on population-level health, hence the need to create quality appraisal tools that inform the reader about how well the trial was done. In Psychology, I rarely have discussions about the overall study quality of a psychology study, and when I do, these usually relate to randomisation and blinding—issues that psychologists are acutely aware of as methods to address important sources of bias in experimental studies.

By contrast, in the land of survey study designs, psychologists tend to focus their efforts on using the best quality measures, in terms of reliability (and sometimes validity), and keeping attrition low if using a prospective/longitudinal study design, but otherwise seem happy to carry on as if study quality does not apply to them. Looking back at my previous survey studies, issues of reliability and sample attrition are the only consistent indices of study quality mentioned in the papers. Indeed, if you had asked me to rate the study quality of the papers in my first three meta-analyses (Cooke et al., 2016; Cooke & French, 2008; Cooke & Sheeran, 2004), I would not have known where to start, although, in Cooke et al. (2016), we did exclude a paper because we judged it to use an invalid measure of a construct.

Since completing Cooke et al. (2016), Protogerou and Hagger's (2020) Quality of Survey Studies in Psychology (Q-SSP) tool has been published. This tool can be used to judge the quality of survey studies. My Professional Doctorate in Health Psychology student, Amina Saadi, used this tool in her systematic review of predictors of influenza vaccine uptake in hospital-based healthcare workers, and found it to be a really effective way to judge the quality of correlational studies. As with the Cochrane Risk of Bias tool criteria, Amina found in her included studies that there were several criteria that authors did not routinely address: reporting of sample demographics, psychometric properties of measures, and operational definitions of the focal behaviour (vaccine uptake). Hopefully, over time psychologists will become more familiar with this tool and this will improve the standard of both research design, using the tool to ensure that correlational studies follow best practice in study design, and the reporting of information. I will use this tool the next time I run a meta-analysis of correlations.

Summary

The aim of this chapter was to get you thinking about quality appraisal for meta-analysis. Initially, I did this by talking about different biases that affect perceptions of study quality. I then provided an example of how to quality appraise a study using an experimental study design and offered advice for correlational study designs. I'll end with a couple of top tips for quality appraisal:

- Read and re-read your papers multiple times to check you have the correct methodological information when quality appraising your studies. Relative to other disciplines, psychology studies often fail to provide as much detail on criteria, including allocation concealment and selective reporting, so you are going to have to infer what happened (helpfully, psychologists are generally pretty awesome at inference, as we do it all the time).
- Ask a review buddy to independently quality appraise all included studies. This might sound like a lot of work, but it is a good way to ensure you've both reached the same inference.
- Keep a folder of quality appraisal forms for easy access to information when you are interpreting results of your meta-analysis (especially moderator analyses).

References

Chambers, C. (2017). *The seven deadly sins of psychology: A manifesto for reforming the culture of scientific practice*. Princeton University Press.

Cooke, R., Dahdah, M., Norman, P., & French, D. P. (2016). How well does the theory of planned behaviour predict alcohol consumption? A systematic review and meta-analysis. *Health Psychology Review, 10*, 148–167. https://doi.org/10.1080/17437199.2014.947547

Cooke, R., & French, D. P. (2008). How well do the theory of reasoned action and theory of planned behaviour predict intentions and attendance at screening programmes? A meta-analysis. *Psychology & Health, 23*(7), 745–765. https://doi.org/10.1080/08870440701544437

Cooke, R., McEwan, H., & Norman, P. (2023). The effect of forming implementation intentions on alcohol consumption: A systematic review and meta-analysis. *Drug and Alcohol Review, 42*, 68–80. https://doi.org/10.1111/dar.13553

Cooke, R., & Sheeran, P. (2004). Moderation of cognition-intention and cognition-behaviour relations: A meta-analysis of properties of variables from the theory of planned behaviour. *The British Journal of Social Psychology, 43*(Pt 2), 159–186. https://doi.org/10.1348/0144666041501688

Cooke, R., Trebachzyk, H., Harris, P., & Wright, A. J. (2014). Self-affirmation promotes physical activity. *Journal of Sport and Exercise Psychology, 36*(2), 217–223. https://doi.org/10.1123/jsep.2013-0041

Higgins, J. P. T., & Green, S. (2011). *Cochrane handbook for systematic reviews of interventions. The Cochrane*. Collaboration.

Protogerou, C., & Hagger, M. S. (2020). A checklist to assess the quality of survey studies in psychology. *Methods in Psychology, 3*, 100031. https://doi.org/10.1016/j.metip.2020.100031

Radtke, T., Ostergaard, M., Cooke, R., & Scholz, U. (2017). Web-based alcohol intervention: Study of systematic attrition of heavy drinkers. *Journal of Medical Internet Research, 19*(6), e217. https://doi.org/10.2196/jmir.6780

Wittleder, S., Kappes, A., Oettingen, G., Gollwitzer, P. M., Jay, M., & Morgenstern, J. (2019). Mental contrasting with implementation intentions reduces drinking when drinking is hazardous: An online self-regulation intervention. *Health Education & Behavior, 46*(4), 666–676. https://doi.org/10.1177/1090198119826284

Data Synthesis for Meta-Analysis 7

Meta-Analysis Is a Form of Data Synthesis

An essential difference between conducting a meta-analysis and running a systematic review is how you synthesise the data you have extracted from studies. In a meta-analysis, data synthesis always involves pooling (synthesising) effect sizes. While some systematic reviews include meta-analyses, it is not the case in others. It depends on studies included in the review. For example, if you are running a systematic review of RCTs, then a meta-analysis is often possible because RCTs necessarily look for differences between two groups on an outcome(s), allowing you to calculate effect size differences or other summary statistics like odds ratios, risk ratios, relative risks used in medicine. In contrast, when running a systematic review of psychology studies, these often use a range of study designs, or have heterogeneity in outcome measures, meaning a meta-analysis might not be possible.

Returning to meta-analysis, you are aiming to produce a precise estimate of the overall effect size statistic of interest; in Cooke et al. (2016), we wanted to precisely estimate the correlations for theory of planned behaviour relationships in alcohol studies; in Cooke et al. (2023), we wanted to precisely estimate the effect size difference in weekly alcohol use and heavy episodic drinking for drinkers asked to form vs not form implementation intentions. To achieve both goals, we focused on statistical information reported by the included studies. Indeed, we had to exclude several studies in each meta due to a lack of statistical information. This is one reason that meta-analyses often have a smaller number of included studies than a systematic review of the same topic; no effect sizes means no meta-analysis.

R. Cooke, *Meta-Analysis for Psychologists*,
https://doi.org/10.1007/978-3-031-73773-2_7

Comparing Oranges to Apples, and Why This Matters for Data Synthesis

A common metaphor used when discussing meta-analysis is to avoid comparing oranges to apples, in other words, how similar are the included studies to one another? There are many dimensions on which to consider studies as similar or different. One dimension is sample characteristics. For instance, in Cooke et al. (2016), we found that 31 of our 33 studies recruited samples where more than 50% of the sample identified as female. Alternatively, in Cooke et al. (2023), we found that some studies recruited from universities while others recruited from community settings. We ran moderator analyses (see Chap. 12) that showed implementation intentions were more effective at reducing weekly alcohol use in community versus university student samples.

Although it's important to think about sample characteristics when considering studies as similar or different to one another, I think it is even more important to consider methodological issues when comparing studies. For example, did the included studies all use similar measures of psychological variables or similar measures of outcomes? I'll give an example from Cooke et al. (2016) to cover correlations and Cooke et al. (2023) to cover effect size differences to highlight that the type of meta-analysis you run can affect how this issue is considered.

In Cooke et al. (2016), we were interested in relationships between theory of planned behaviour constructs, for example, attitudes, subjective norms, perceived behavioural control, and outcomes, for example, intentions, drinking behaviour. In most of the included studies, authors reported that they had developed items to assess theory of planned behaviour constructs either following Ajzen's recommendations or adapted items that were already published based on these recommendations. Reporting either approach satisfied the review team because they indicated following an agreed process for item development or adaptation that ensured items reflected the latent constructs being measured. However, there was one paper we excluded at the full-text stage because of how they measured perceived behavioural control. In this paper, the authors used a validated measure of alcohol problems as an index of control. While we thought you *could* indirectly infer that reporting more alcohol problems indicates lower control over drinking, we decided to exclude this paper because all the other studies had measured perceived behaviour control either following Ajzen's recommendations or using items that had been developed following recommendations. While it might seem harsh to exclude results from the paper on this basis, as the goal of meta-analysis is to produce a precise estimate of an effect size, in this case, the correlation between perceived control and intentions, we decided it would be better to exclude that paper as it differed from the other papers we included.

Of course, sometimes you must be more flexible in decisions about which effect sizes to include. In Cooke et al. (2016), we had a wide range of measures of one outcome: drinking behaviour. There was no way that we could exclude papers due to variation in measures of drinking behaviour, in the way we excluded the paper for measuring perceived behavioural control differently. In some ways, the differences in how we treated variability in measures of constructs and outcomes reflect the reality that there is more homogeneity in measures of constructs than outcomes. Indeed, we did acknowledged heterogeneity in drinking behaviour measures in the paper, going so far as to create a five-category coding scheme to classify papers and using moderator analyses to compare results. The heterogeneity in how drinking behaviour was measured allowed us to see if effect sizes for different behavioural measures varied depending on how behaviour was measured. Conversely, homogeneity in the measures of perceived behavioural control meant we could not do the same and led to the exclusion of that paper.

Moving from correlations to effect size differences, you need to think about the outcome measures very carefully. In Cooke et al. (2023), for example, there was one study that measured heavy episodic drinking using a scale, while all other studies measured frequency of heavy episodic drinking using absolute values (i.e. zero times, three times). After some lively debates with my co-author, I decided to exclude this paper from the heavy episodic drinking analysis because, from my perspective, measuring behaviour on a scale is different to measuring behaviour in absolute values. Including both types of measure in the same meta-analysis is like comparing an orange to an apple. One approach you can take before excluding papers is to run a sensitivity analysis; this is where you run the meta-analysis multiple times, each time removing one effect size, to see if the overall effect size is sensitive to the absence of any effect size.

In sum, I wanted to highlight the issue of comparing oranges with apples at this point, before you run meta-analysis, as in all the work that goes into screening, data extraction, and quality appraisal, it is sometimes missed that you only think about the comparability of studies near the end of the process of preparing data for synthesis. Next, I will revisit some of the information on effect sizes presented in Chap. 3.

Thinking About Correlations' Direction and Magnitude

A key part of any meta-analysis is interpreting effect sizes from included studies. You need to reflect on the direction and magnitude of each effect size because understanding the results for each included study will help you interpret the overall effect size produced by meta-analysis. The more you practise interpretation of effect sizes in terms of direction and magnitude, the easier you will find it to interpret meta-analytic results, which involves the same task based on pooling across studies.

I've included Table 7.1 to help you practise these ideas. This table contains data from ten imaginary studies that have correlated drinking intentions (i.e. plans to drink in the future) and drinking behaviour (i.e. self-reported alcohol consumption) measured between one week and four weeks later (i.e. using a prospective design). You can infer quite a lot of important information from each row without running a meta-analysis: You can note their directions (positive; negative; null) and their magnitudes (small; medium; large) using Cohen's (1992) guidelines (see Chap. 3).

Start with a simple question—"Are all the correlations in the same direction?" In our case the answer is "yes" —they are all positive correlations; having higher drinking intentions is correlated with more self-reported drinking behaviour. This

Table 7.1 Example table of correlations between drinking intentions and behaviour

Study authors + year	Correlation (*r*)
Arking and Jones (2010)	0.25
Biggs and Smith (2002)	0.54
Cole et al. (2015)	0.45
David et al. (2018)	0.35
Erasmus et al. (2009)	0.70
Feely and Touchy (2007)	0.65
Gent et al. (2020)	0.30
Horseham and Smooth (2021)	0.40
Illy et al. (2013)	0.60
Jacobi and Jordan (2014)	0.65

uniformity of direction means that when we run the meta-analysis, we should expect to find a positive overall correlation (i.e. the correlation based on pooling results across studies), if we don't, it's likely we've done something wrong!

We can also think about what these positive correlations mean and whether this fits in with what you expect in terms of theory. Results match Cooke et al. (2016), where we had positive correlations between drinking intentions and behaviour for 19 studies using prospective designs. When running statistical tests, always remember that statistics are there to help you answer a question—is what I expect to happen happening? Interpreting results can be challenging, so I recommend before you start, remind yourself what you are doing, for example, what variables are you correlating with one another, and why that is interesting to you. Thinking about these non-statistical questions will help you when it comes to interpreting or inferring results because they prime you to know what to look for.

How about magnitude? "Do all the correlations have the same magnitude?" In our case, the answer to the question is "no"—correlations vary in magnitude. Using Cohen's (1992) guidelines (see Chap. 3), we have one small correlation, four medium correlations, and five large correlations. The lack of uniformity in magnitude means we are uncertain about the size of the overall correlation, but you can make an educated guess that because 9/10 correlations are either medium or large-sized then the overall correlation is likely to be either medium or large-sized.

Answering these two questions about direction and magnitude of individual study effect sizes primes you for your meta-analysis because we already know that we need to focus more on magnitude and less on direction, when interpreting our results; all correlations are positive, meaning that as intentions to drink increase, so does drinking behaviour. Having covered inference of direction and magnitude for a set of correlations, let's do the same for effect size differences.

Thinking About Effect Size Differences Direction and Magnitude

The same process of inference of direction and magnitude is also possible for effect size differences. Table 7.2 includes statistics from ten imaginary studies reporting effect size differences for adolescents receiving vs not receiving a behaviour change

Table 7.2 Example table of effect size differences for a behaviour change intervention to reduce screen time

Authors	Effect size difference (*d*)
Keane et al. (2002)	0.20
Linus et al. (1999)	0.59
Mimms et al. (1977)	0.70
Noone et al. (1985)	0.64
Owen (2023)	0.75
Peeps et al. (2015)	0.39
Quest et al. (2016)	0.22
Ricki et al. (2007)	0.47
Sopp et al. (2012)	0.44
Tapp et al. (2003)	0.78

intervention to reduce screen time. As before, you can note down the direction and magnitude of these effect sizes before you run any data synthesis.

Let's think about direction first: "Are all the effect size differences in the same direction?" In this case the answer is "yes". In each study, there is a positive effect size difference, that is, where the intervention group reduced their screen time more than the control group. So, there is uniformity in direction for this set of effect size differences. How about magnitude? Using Cohen's (1992) guidelines, we have five medium effect size differences and five small effect size differences. The skills you've just practised are the same ones you will need when interpreting what the output of your meta-analysis is. The only difference is that you will be interpreting the direction and magnitude of the overall effect size rather than the individual effect sizes shown in Tables 7.1 and 7.2.

What Statistical Information Does Meta-Analysis Produce?

Meta-analysis outputs statistical information that relates to three key points of interest. First, meta-analysis produces a sample-weighted average effect size, that is, a sample-weighted average correlation between two variables or a sample-weighted average effect size difference between two groups on an outcome. Meta-analysis provides the average effect size (correlation or effect size difference) across included studies after weighting each individual effect size by sample size; studies with larger sample sizes are given greater weight, hence the phrase sample-weighted. Meta-analysis will also output statistics that you can use to infer the significance of the sample-weighted statistic you are interested in. I will talk more about these values in Chaps. 9 and 10 and weighting in Chap. 11. Second, meta-analysis produces statistics that indicate the extent of heterogeneity among the effect sizes in your included studies. Meta-analysis provides statistics that tell you if the studies' effect sizes differ from one another (heterogeneity) or if they are similar (homogeneity). We'll talk about ways to deal with this issue using moderation in Chap. 12. Third, meta-analysis outputs statistics to help clarify if there is evidence of publication bias in the included studies. Meta-analysis allows researchers to compare effect sizes from included studies to see if they represent the full range of potential values or if they only represent a narrow range of potential values, usually positive, that suggest that only positive effects are published. Chapter 13 will go over publication bias in more detail. Let's work through each of these ideas—sample-weighting, heterogeneity, publication bias—one by one.

What Does Sample-Weighting Mean?

The first point I mentioned in the previous paragraph was about sample-weighting. Table 7.3 contains the same imaginary studies as Table 7.1 but with sample sizes added, which range from 50 to 2000. In Chap. 3, we discussed the idea that we should put more weight (importance) on effect sizes from studies based on larger samples, because these results are more likely to reflect the population effect size than equivalent effect sizes from smaller samples. In effect, meta-analysis outputs an estimate of the population effect size—this is the sample-weighted average correlation or the sample-weighted average effect size difference.

You can ask the question of studies in Table 7.3—"Which study is most likely to represent the population effect size (e.g. correlation between drinking intentions and self-reported drinking behaviour)?" The answer is Cole et al. (2000). Why? This correlation is based on the largest sample size ($N = 2000$) and so is most likely to reflect the population correlation between drinking intentions and behaviour. You can turn the question around and ask, "Which study is least likely to represent the population effect size?" This time the answer is Jacobi and Jordan (2014). A sample of $N = 50$ does not inspire much confidence that results reflect the population correlation. In your own meta-analysis, the sample sizes might vary from this example, but the logic underpinning my reasoning will always be the same; the study with the largest sample size (even if it does not look very large!) will ALWAYS be given the

Table 7.3 Example table of correlations between drinking intentions and behaviour with sample sizes

Study authors + year	Correlation (r)	Sample size (N)
Arking and Jones (2010)	0.25	100
Biggs and Smith (2002)	0.54	200
Cole et al. (2015)	0.45	2000
David et al. (2018)	0.35	150
Erasmus et al. (2009)	0.70	75
Feely and Touchy (2007)	0.65	400
Gent et al. (2020)	0.30	475
Horseham and Smooth (2021)	0.40	150
Illy et al. (2013)	0.60	125
Jacobi and Jordan (2014)	0.65	50

most weight in a meta-analysis. Equally, the study with smallest sample size (even if it does not look very small!) will ALWAYS be given the least weight in a meta-analysis.

So, even before you run a meta-analysis, you can make the following inferences about the correlations and sample sizes reported in this set of studies:

- Correlations are all in the same *direction* (positive).
- Correlations vary in *magnitude* (from small ($r = 0.25$) to large ($r = 0.70$).
- Sample sizes vary from 50 to 2000 participants, with most studies recruiting at least 100 participants.

There's one final inference you could potentially make; it's highly likely that all these correlations are significantly different from zero (i.e. a correlation of $r = 0.00$). Because the smallest correlation is $r = 0.25$, which is quite far from $r = 0.00$, I think it's a fairly safe bet that all our correlations are significantly different from zero. However, the beauty of meta-analysis is that you don't need to take that bet in ignorance. By running the meta-analysis of these studies (see Chap. 9) you'll know for sure!

I've added the sample sizes for the imaginary studies in Tables 7.2 to Table 7.4. A key difference here is that you have separate sample sizes for control and intervention groups, rather than the overall sample you get with a correlation. This is because with correlations, you are running a test of association, and average results across the whole sample, whereas with an effect size difference, you are running a test of difference and want to maintain separation between the groups. The idea, nevertheless, remains the same; effect size differences based on more people are assigned greater weight (importance) in meta-analysis relative to studies based on fewer people. Adapting our question about confidence in effect sizes to the studies in Table 6.4, based on sample size, we should have greatest confidence that results from Peeps et al. (2015), with a total sample size of $N = 950$, represent the population effect size difference and least confidence in Quest et al.'s (2016) results, with a total sample size of $N = 35$, represent the population effect size difference. The rule of thumb is more people = more confidence, although this does depend somewhat on the numbers of participants in each group.

I will finish off this section by reminding you of the inferences you can make about studies in Table 7.4:

- Effect size differences are in the same direction (favour experimental group).
- Effect size differences vary in magnitude (from medium ($d = 0.67$) to large ($d = 5.86$).
- (Total) Sample sizes vary from $N = 35$ to $N = 950$.

Unlike the correlations, I am not prepared to make the inference that all these effect size differences are significantly different from zero. Quest et al.'s (2016) results, which combine the smallest effect size difference ($d = 0.22$) with the

Table 7.4 Example table of effect size differences for a behaviour change intervention to reduce screen time with sample sizes

Authors	Effect size difference (*d*)	Control group sample size (*N*)	Experimental group sample size (*N*)
Keane et al. (2002)	0.20	50	50
Linus et al. (1999)	0.59	75	75
Mimms et al. (1977)	0.70	25	25
Noone et al. (1985)	0.64	125	120
Owen (2023)	0.75	250	200
Peeps et al. (2015)	0.39	500	450
Quest et al. (2016)	0.22	15	20
Ricki et al. (2007)	0.47	115	120
Sopp et al. (2012)	0.44	55	45
Tapp et al. (2003)	0.78	30	20

smallest total sample size ($N = 35$), make me pause before claiming that result is significantly different from zero. We'll pick up these ideas in more detail in Chap. 10. Let's move on to talking about heterogeneity of effect sizes.

What Does Heterogeneity of Effect Sizes Mean?

As a psychologist, you will have undoubtedly come across the concepts of homogeneity and heterogeneity before. Think back to classes on ANOVA or t-tests and the homogeneity of variances tests you ran. We can use this principle to help us understand the statistics we use in meta-analysis. We've already discussed that the effect sizes in Table 7.1 varied in their magnitude; some correlations were small, some medium, and some large. The original goal of meta-analysis was to produce an overall (sample-weighted) average effect size that represents data from a set of studies that is homogeneous, the idea being that this overall effect size would provide a sufficiently precise estimate for use by researchers. I've yet to run a meta-analysis where the effect sizes for the overall analysis are homogeneous except when most studies have null effects!!! I think this is probably a function of meta-analysing psychology studies, which contain many sources of differences between studies. In short, we're not great at standardising our research methods (especially the measures we use) relative to other disciplines. Psychology studies often recruit small sample sizes, which can lead to volatility in results between studies. How can meta-analysis help us to work out the extent of heterogeneity between studies? In two ways: using statistics to calculate the extent of heterogeneity, and by creating forest plots to visualise the effect sizes from our included studies.

Two main statistics that meta-analysts report when describing the heterogeneity of their effect sizes are: the *Q* test (a Chi-square test) and the I^2 index. The *Q* test is like many statistical tests. It takes observed values you have in your dataset and tests the idea that they significantly differ from the expected value. This expectation makes intuitive sense; in meta-analysis, you are aiming to pool together statistics from studies that have done pretty much the same thing, like correlate drinking intentions with drinking behaviour using prospective designs or evaluate the effectiveness of an intervention to reduce screen time. Despite this aim, most of the times I've run *Q* tests have produced significant effects, which mean that data are heterogeneous. We'll return to discuss homogeneity in Chap. 12.

The I^2 index (Higgins, 2003) estimates the amount of variability in study results that is due to real differences between the studies, rather than chance. So, if you have an I^2 value of 50% that means 50% of variation in results is due to differences between the studies. I^2 values of 25%, 50%, and 75% have been proposed by Higgins (2003) as indicative of low, medium, and high heterogeneity in results between studies.

While the *Q* test and I^2 index give you a sense of the heterogeneity of the effect sizes, I find forest plots are really helpful in unpicking what is causing heterogeneity in effect sizes. A forest plot (see Figs. 2.1, 9.5, or 10.5) allows the reader to quickly determine the pattern of results, that is, are studies roughly similar or do they differ from one another, as well as helping you to spot outliers, whether they are reporting larger, or smaller, effect sizes than the other studies. We'll return to this issue in Part III of the book. Next, we'll cover publication bias statistics and funnel plots.

How Do You Identify Publication Bias in Meta-Analysis?

As discussed in Chap. 2, publication bias is a key issue in research, especially in psychology, where we have lived through the replication crisis. We'll go on to discuss publication bias in depth in Chap. 13, so here I'll restrict myself to talking about how meta-analysis allows you to identify publication bias. Indeed, meta-analysis is particularly well suited to this task.

Meta-analysis outputs several statistical indicators of publication bias, including the Fail Safe N values, Rank correlation, and regression tests as well as funnel plots and trim and fill statistics. I briefly introduce these statistics and talk about funnel plots now before talk in later chapters (see Chaps. 9, 10, and 13).

Fail-Safe *N* values (Orwin, 1983; Rosenthal, 1979) quantify how many studies with *null* effect sizes (i.e. $d = 0.00$ or $r = 0.00$) you would need to find to undermine confidence in your results. Often Fail-Safe N values are well into the 1000s, based on data from 20 or 30 studies. As it's unlikely that you have failed to locate 1000 studies that ALL have null effect sizes, you can indirectly infer confidence in your results. In terms of publication bias, a small fail-safe value, like a value of 2 or 3 studies based on following a meta-analysis of results from 15 studies, could indicate publication bias, as it suggests you only needed to include a couple of additional studies to undermine confidence in your results.

Other statistical tests look for asymmetry in effect sizes as a marker of publication bias. For instance, Egger et al.'s (1997) regression test checks if the effect sizes in your meta-analysis are asymmetrical or not, that is, is the spread of effect sizes broadly symmetrical or broadly asymmetrical? A significant result means you have an asymmetrical distribution that may be missing negative (or null) effect sizes that did not get published. Meta-analysis also outputs Duval and Tweedie's trim and fill statistic (Duval & Tweedie, 2000a, 2000b), which tells you how many missing studies there 'should' be, that is, assuming a symmetrical distribution of effect sizes, and will adjust the overall effect size to account for these missing studies.

What do I mean by asymmetry in a set of effect sizes? Well, all else being equal, we should expect the effect sizes we include in our meta-analysis to reflect a spread of values, some above the overall effect size and some below, because the overall effect size is an average. If there's no publication bias, you should have a (roughly) similar number of effect sizes above and below the overall effect size AND you should have a similar number of studies with small sample sizes showing positive effects as show negative or null effect sizes. If this happens, you have a symmetrical distribution, with results either side of the overall effect size (see Figs. 8.9 or 9.9 for examples of funnel plots showing symmetrical distributions).

In contrast to symmetrical distributions, what happens with publication bias is that studies with small sample sizes AND significant effect sizes are more likely to be published than similar studies with small sample sizes AND non-significant effect sizes. This favouring of significant effect sizes with small sample sizes undermines the symmetry of your plot, implying that you are missing some studies.

Judging the asymmetry of your effect size is best done by checking your statistics and inspecting a funnel plot, which provides a visualisation of effect sizes by plotting the effect size for each study on the x axis and the standard error of the effect size on the y axis. Funnel plots help us to identify asymmetry in effect sizes by taking advantage of the fact that the larger the sample size, the smaller the standard error an effect size has; a standard error is a measure of dispersion for a population in a similar way to a standard deviation is a measure of dispersion for a sample. So, a funnel plot takes this idea—larger samples = smaller standard errors—and plots the effect sizes against the standard errors to highlight studies that have larger sample errors (suggesting small samples) and significant effect sizes.

Doing this allows you to see if there are any studies that fall outside of the funnel—typically these have medium or large effect sizes but also larger standard errors, at least in relation to the other studies included in the meta-analysis. You will see these studies at the bottom of the funnel plot, where the funnel is wider, because the y axis is scaled so that larger standard errors (i.e. those studies with smaller sample sizes) are at the bottom of the y axis. Some researchers advise to look at the bottom of the plot for the presence of studies that appear to the right of the overall effect size (indicating higher effect size than the average) but also near the bottom of plot (indicating small sample sizes). Having checked for the presence of these types of studies (positive effects based on small samples) you can then scan left and look for equivalent studies to the left of the overall effect size (negative, or null, effects based on small samples). If you find there're few or zero studies on the left of the plot near the bottom, you might have evidence of publication bias. We'll come back to this issue when we run meta-analyses in Chaps. 9 and 10 and in depth in Chap. 13.

Summary

This chapter has focused on reiterating how to interpret effect sizes as well as priming you for the three key bits of information you'll generate in your jamovi output: the overall effect size; the extent of heterogeneity in effect sizes; evidence of publication bias. In Chap. 8, we'll go over the practical aspects of installing jamovi and major to run meta-analyses before outlining how to run a meta-analysis of correlations in Chap. 9 and meta-analysis of effect size differences in Chap. 10. The tasks below are included to help you practise applying the principles of interpreting effect sizes in terms of direction and magnitude covered in this chapter.

Tasks

1. Complete Table 7.5 by writing in the direction and magnitude of each effect size (Hint: Use Cohen's (1992) guidelines, reported in Chap. 3, to infer the magnitude).
2. Complete Table 7.6 by writing in the direction and magnitude of each effect size (Hint: Use Cohen's (1992) guidelines, reported in Chap. 3, to infer the magnitude).
3. Table 7.7 includes a set of results for eight studies that reported effect size differences for an experimental manipulation testing the effects of using gain vs loss frames to encourage physical activity: Gain frames are messages that emphasise the gains that follow behaviour change (i.e. what you will gain by being more

Table 7.5 Correlations between perceived behavioural control over drinking and drinking intentions

Study names	Correlation (r)	N	Direction	Magnitude
Arking and Jones (2010)	0.25	150		
Biggs and Smith (2002)	−0.02	200		
Cole et al. (2015)	0.10	350		
David et al. (2018)	0.35	35		
Erasmus et al. (2009)	−0.50	180		
Feely and Touchy (2007)	0.45	389		
Gent et al. (2020)	0.14	100		
Horseham and Smooth (2021)	0.00	80		
Illy et al. (2013)	−0.15	125		
Jacobi and Jordan (2014)	0.55	165		

Table 7.6 Example table of effect size differences for a behaviour change intervention to increase digital resilience skills with sample sizes

Authors	Effect size difference (*d*)	Direction	Magnitude
Keane et al. (2002)	0.50		
Linus et al. (1999)	0.35		
Mimms et al. (1977)	0.80		
Noone et al. (1985)	0.00		
Owen (2023)	0.15		
Peeps et al. (2015)	0.20		
Quest et al. (2016)	−0.45		
Ricki et al. (2007)	0.75		
Sopp et al. (2012)	0.15		
Tapp et al. (2003)	0.25		

Table 7.7 Example table of effect size differences for gains versus loss frame messages to increase physical activity

Authors	Effect size difference (*d*)	Direction	Magnitude
Erikson (2002)	−0.22		
Maldini (1999)	0.37		
Gower et al. (1977)	−0.80		
Gatting (1985)	0.00		
Montana and Young (2023)	0.12		
Rodgers (2015)	0.29		
Smith (2016)	−0.54		
Backley (2007)	−0.75		
Maresca et al. (2024)	0.05		
Frank (2003)	−0.08		

physically active). Loss frames are messages that emphasise the losses that follow failure to change behaviour (i.e. what you lose by being physically inactive). Complete Table 7.7 by writing the direction and magnitude of each effect size (Hint: Use Cohen's (1992) guidelines, reported in Chap. 3, to infer the magnitude).

References

Cohen, J. (1992). A power primer. *Psychological Bulletin, 112*(1), 155–159.

Cooke, R., Dahdah, M., Norman, P., & French, D. P. (2016). How well does the theory of planned behaviour predict alcohol consumption? A systematic review and meta-analysis. *Health Psychology Review, 10*, 148–167. https://doi.org/10.1080/17437199.2014.947547

Cooke, R., McEwan, H., & Norman, P. (2023). The effect of forming implementation intentions on alcohol consumption: A systematic review and meta-analysis. *Drug and Alcohol Review, 42*, 68–80. https://doi.org/10.1111/dar.13553

Duval, S., & Tweedie, R. (2000a). A nonparametric 'trim and fill' method of accounting for publication bias in meta-analysis. *Journal of the American Statistical Association, 95*, 89–98.

Duval, S., & Tweedie, R. (2000b). Trim and fill: A simple funnel-plot-based method of testing and adjusting for publication bias in meta-analysis. *Biometrics, 56*, 455–463.

Egger, M., Higgins, J. P. T., & Smith, D. (1997). Bias in meta-analysis detected by a simple, graphical test. *BMJ, 315*, 629–634.

Higgins, J. P. T. (2003). Measuring inconsistency in meta-analyses. *BMJ, 327*(7414), 557–560. https://doi.org/10.1136/bmj.327.7414.557

Orwin, R. G. (1983). A fail-safe *N* for effect size in meta-analysis. *Journal of Educational Statistics, 8*(2), 157–159. https://doi.org/10.3102/10769986008002157

Rosenthal, R. R. (1979). The File drawer problem and tolerance for null results. *Psychological Bulletin, 86*, 638–641.

Part III

Conducting Meta-Analysis in Jamovi

8 Using jamovi to Conduct Meta-Analyses

A Lucky Introduction to jamovi

In October 2017, I attended a lunchtime seminar at Aston University delivered by postdoctoral student Dr Sam Nash. Sam wanted to let staff know about two new statistical software packages, jamovi and JASP, that ran code from the open-source platform R. Like most UK psychologists, I had been taught to use SPSS as an undergraduate and despite some qualms about this programme, including endless output files and ugly graphs, I had stuck with it through completion of my PhD and into years of teaching statistics because the alternatives did not seem appealing; the open software platform R seemed very powerful but brought back memories of the 'good' (bad) days of me spending hours writing SPSS syntax files during my PhD. We did not have a licence for STATA, so there was little point in learning how to use that programme.

Sam's presentation was pretty much perfect for me—here were two free packages that ran R using an SPSS-like interface. Happy days! After downloading the packages I had a quick play with some data and was blown away. Here were intuitive programmes that eliminated SPSS' key weaknesses with output and graphs. For instance, R is known to produce beautiful graphs and so jamovi and JASP graphs are beautiful too. I liked the fact that you could have the output file overlap with the data file, something that is more useful than it sounds, and really liked that once you had run an analysis you could tailor the output by either adding or removing information. No longer would I have to scroll through endless pages of irrelevant statistics to find what I needed, brilliant! The cherry on the cake was the discovery that jamovi would output effect size differences for *t*-tests, something that SPSS had not learned how to do at that point in time. Finally, I was delighted to see that both jamovi and JASP had an option to run meta-analysis.

Since those early days learning about jamovi and JASP, I have used both when teaching psychology postgraduate statistics. One class from my time teaching MSc Research Methods students at the University of Liverpool stayed with me. I asked

R. Cooke, *Meta-Analysis for Psychologists*,
https://doi.org/10.1007/978-3-031-73773-2_8

them to run analyses in SPSS, which they knew from their undergraduate degree, and then again in jamovi, which was new to them. The feedback from the students was unlike anything I experienced teaching stats before—they thanked me for introducing them to jamovi! One student even asked why we still taught statistical analysis using SPSS??!

Why This Book Uses jamovi to Run Meta-Analyses

Discovering that both jamovi and JASP had an option to run meta-analysis piqued my interest as, throughout my career, I had always used stand-alone packages to complete meta-analyses; I was taught meta-analysis using Ralf Schwarzer's (1988) Meta programme, a DOS programme that did a pretty good job before Windows Vista killed it off. You can still download Ralf's software at http://userpage.fu-berlin.de/~health/meta_e.htm, including the manual which has some useful tips for running meta-analysis. I moved on to using Comprehensive Meta-Analysis (Borenstein et al., 2005) produced by Michael Borenstein and colleagues. CMA is a nice programme with two downsides. First, as licensed software, you must pay for it. Second, CMA is not Mac-friendly. Even if you don't use CMA for your meta-analysis, I recommend reading Borenstein et al.'s (Borenstein et al., 2021) excellent textbook that accompanies the software. It provides in-depth explanation of how meta-analysis works.

So, my choice for this book was between jamovi and JASP. Both are free and Mac-friendly. The main reason I went for jamovi is that it allows you to run meta-analysis by entering data for effect size differences using two methods: (1) entering the mean, standard deviation and sample sizes for the control and experiment/intervention groups or (2) entering the effect sizes and standard errors. In JASP, you must use method (2). I wanted to use a package that let me calculate effect size differences based on method (1) because I know that many psychology papers fail to report effect sizes. By teaching you how to use method (1), I'm aiming to make your life a bit easier as you only need to enter the data reported by the authors—most authors report means and standard deviations, although sometimes authors do report adjusted means, so watch out for that! In sum, jamovi's greater flexibility in how you enter data for meta-analysis persuaded me to use it and this is why I am recommending it for your meta-analysis. The next section will outline how to download and install jamovi.

Downloading and Installing jamovi

First search for 'jamovi download' using any search engine. Then download the version for your type of computer, Windows, Mac, Linux, Chrome. There's a cloud version too, but I am going to stick to the desktop version as this is what I have used for conducting meta-analysis. After downloading, installing, and opening jamovi, it will look like Fig. 8.1.

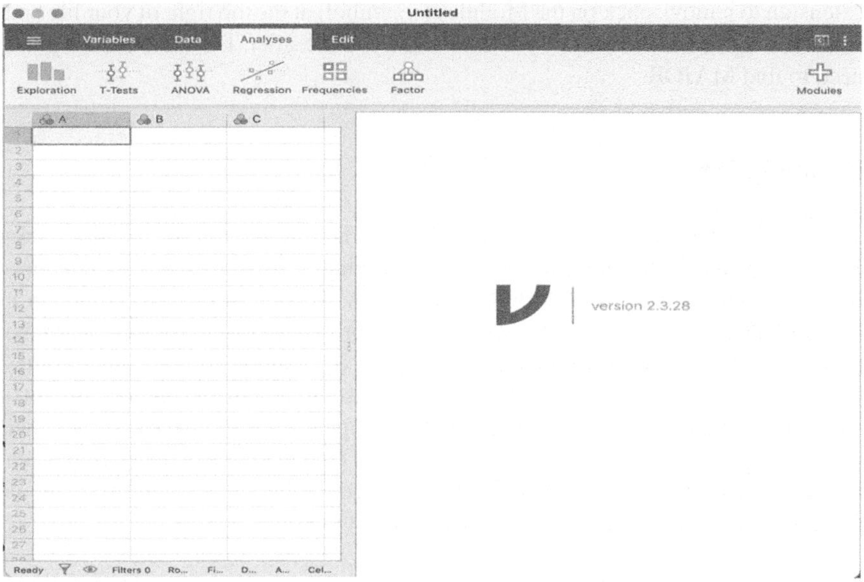

Fig. 8.1 What jamovi looks like when you open it for the first time

You have a data window, where you enter your variables (left-hand side of screenshot, with column headings A B C). Unlike SPSS, jamovi displays the output window alongside the data window (the right-hand side of the screenshot, currently empty because we have not run any analyses). The analysis options on the top bar—Exploration, T-tests, ANOVA, Regression, Frequencies, and Factor—are pre-installed packages. Exploration has descriptive statistics and scatterplots, T-tests contains independent group, paired, one sample. ANOVA has parametric (One way, ANOVA (= multiple factors), Repeated Measures, ANCOVA, and MANCOVA) and non-parametric (Kruskal Wallis, McNemar test) tests. Regression has correlations, partial correlations, linear, logistic regression. Frequencies has binomial test, chi-square goodness of fit and test of association, McNemar test, and log-linear regression. Factor has reliability analysis, exploratory factor analysis, principal components analysis, and confirmatory factor analysis.

Meta-analysis is *not* included as one of the pre-installed options in jamovi. To run meta-analysis, go to the Modules option (top right of screenshot where giant + symbol is).

Modules—A Library of Extensions

A key strength of R is that because it is open source, researchers are free to create updates for it. By installing jamovi, you gain (partial) access to this activity, with new extensions being added to jamovi on a regular basis. If you want to add an extension to jamovi, click on the Modules (+ symbol) at the top right of your file and scroll through the library until you find what you are after. For meta-analysis, we need to find MAJOR.

Installing MAJOR

The MAJOR extension was written by W. Kyle Hamilton to run the metafor package reported in Viechtbauer (2010); metafor provides a set of methods for conducting meta-analysis in R, and MAJOR is the jamovi version of metafor. Although it does not have all the functionality of metafor, it provides enough for us to learn the principles of meta-analysis without all the fun of learning to code (that comes later!). I recommend reading Viechtbauer paper as it will help explain how the software runs and is also a good introduction to principles of meta-analysis. It's another good resource to have as it explains various ways of running meta-analysis and can help expand your knowledge when you've learned the basics. So, your next step is to scroll through the modules until you find MAJOR (see Fig. 8.2).

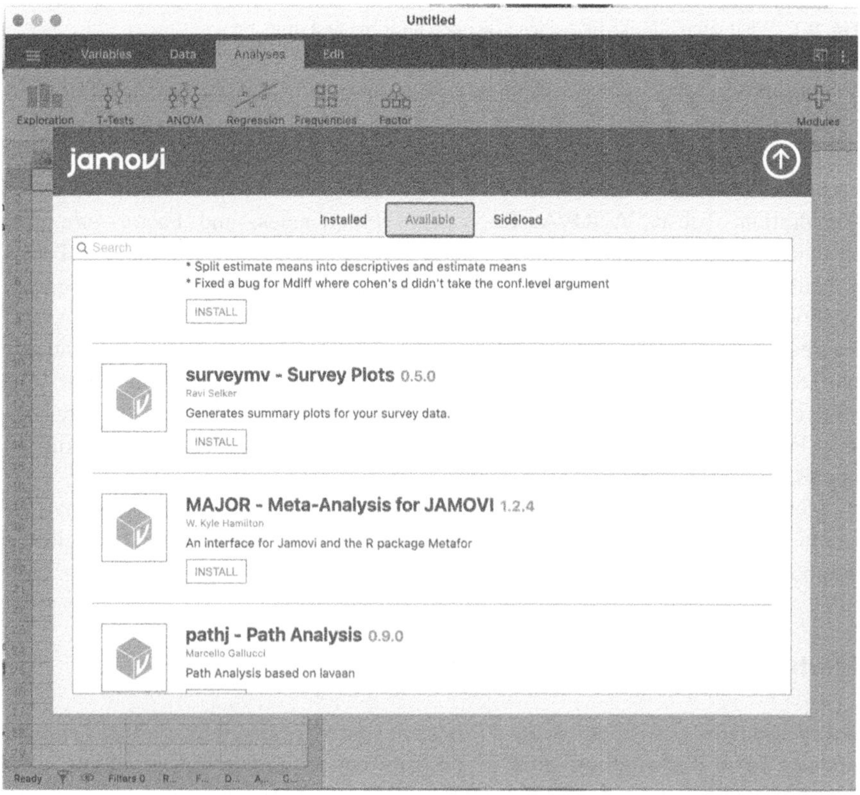

Fig. 8.2 MAJOR in the modules window

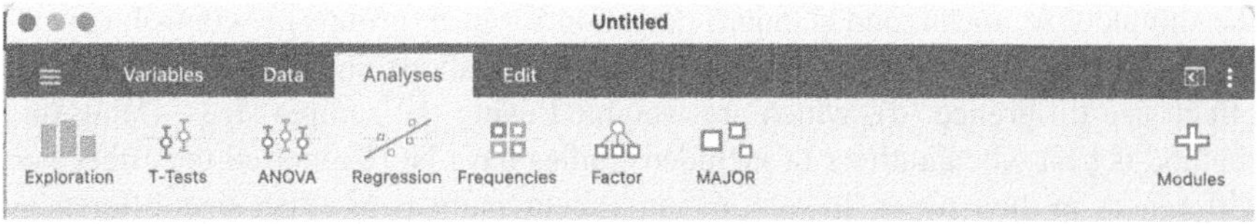

Fig. 8.3 Analyses toolbar in jamovi with MAJOR installed

When you've found it, click on install and you'll notice that MAJOR is now available in your analyses toolbar (see Fig. 8.3).

Setting Up Datasets in jamovi for Using MAJOR

To run a meta-analysis in any software package, you must create a dataset that contains a specific set of variables. In all meta-analytic datasets, you will need a study label/authors variable. For example, in Cooke et al. (2016), we identified included studies based on author and year of publication, for example, Cooke & French (2011). For most studies, this worked fine, but for some we needed to add extra information. For papers that had multiple studies, we labelled these Conner et al. (1999) Study 1, Conner et al. (1999) Study 2, Conner et al. (1999) Study 3.

Alternatively, Zimmermann and Sieverding (2011) reported correlations separately for men and women, so we labelled the results in our dataset as Zimmermann and Sieverding (2011) male and Zimmermann and Sieverding (2011) female. Regardless of the type of meta-analysis you run, MAJOR expects you to have created a variable that serves this function. So, a study label/authors variable is common to all meta-analytic datasets. Other variables included in the dataset depend on whether you are running a meta-analysis of correlations or a meta-analysis of effect size differences.

Creating a Dataset for Meta-Analysis of Correlations

In any meta-analysis of correlations, you need to create a correlation variable (r) and a sample size variable (N): The correlation from each included study is your effect size, and the sample size is used to weight the studies when running the meta-analysis (see Chaps. 3 and 7). Studies with larger sample sizes receive more weighting in sample-weighted average correlations. In sum, to run a meta-analysis of correlations, you need to create three variables: (1) study label/authors; (2) correlation; and (3) sample size.

Creating a Dataset for Meta-Analysis of Effect Size Differences

There are two methods to create a dataset for meta-analysis of effect size differences. Method (1) involves creating a study label/name variable and then entering the sample size, mean, and standard deviation for each group (i.e. control; experimental/intervention). The means and standard deviations are used to generate the effect size difference (d), which are weighted using the sample sizes. Using this method is best when authors of included studies have NOT reported the effect size differences in their paper. In sum, to run a meta-analysis of effect size differences using Method (1), you need to create seven variables: (1) study label/authors; (2) experimental/intervention group mean; (3) experimental/intervention group standard deviation; (4) experimental/intervention group sample size; (5) control group mean; (6) control group standard deviation; and (7) control group sample size.

Method (2) is best used when most of the authors of included studies have reported effect size differences. Using method (2), you only need to create three variables to run a meta-analysis of effect size differences: (1) study label/authors; (2) effect size difference; and (3) standard error or sample variance. You already have the effect size differences so all you need is the standard errors, or sample variances, to allow MAJOR to weight the effect sizes.

I've never been able to run a meta-analysis of effect size differences based on method (2) because the literatures I've meta-analysed to date have failed to include effect size differences in the papers. I thought I should mention it in case you get lucky with your own meta-analysis. As an aside, if most of your studies have reported effect size differences but a couple of studies have not, then I would advise you use either one of the effect size calculators available on the Internet (see Chap. 3) or if you are comfortable with R, download metafor and use the escalc function (see Viechtbauer, 2010, for more information). Either option can be used to calculate the missing d values for you to add to jamovi.

Alternative Software Packages for Running Meta-Analysis

Comprehensive Meta-analysis (CMA: Biostat)

CMA is bespoke software, designed primarily for running meta-analysis. Developed by a team led by Michael Borenstein, it is an easy-to-use package for completing meta-analysis. I used CMA to complete Cooke et al. (2016) and trained the team that ran meta-analyses for Newby et al. (2021) using CMA too. A nice feature of CMA is how well it handles meta-regression, where you are looking at the effects of moderator variables (see Chap. 12). I also like its ability to plot missing studies on funnel plots when you have evidence of publication bias (see Chap. 13). The two main two reasons I do not use CMA any more are (1) CMA does not run on Mac and (2) my licence expired. If you use a PC, do give the trial version of CMA a go to see what you think. It's a viable option for meta-analysis if you have funding to pay for a licence. Another thing in CMA's favour is that it is supported by Borenstein et al. (2021), which provides excellent examples to help learn about meta-analysis.

metafor (Viechtbauer, 2010, within R/R Studio)

metafor, developed by Wolfgang Viechtbauer (2010), is an excellent package for running meta-analyses in R. The MAJOR plugin in jamovi runs metafor in the background. My main reservation with recommending learning about meta-analysis using metafor has nothing to do with the package itself, instead reflecting my belief that many psychology students and psychologists are wary of using R due to it being a code-based programme. Nevertheless, most meta-analysts will ultimately want to migrate from MAJOR to metafor as it has greater functionality, including the helpful escalc function that will generate effect sizes for you, and the possibility of running mixed effects meta-analysis with more than one moderator (see Chap. 12). I used metafor when completing meta-analyses for Cooke et al. (2023).

Summary

In this chapter, I have provided guidance on how to download and install jamovi, how to install MAJOR, as well as information about how to prepare the dataset for meta-analysis. In Chaps. 9 and 10, I will describe how to perform meta-analysis using MAJOR in jamovi. The two tasks are designed to help prepare you for this task.

Tasks

Task 1. Create a dataset for a meta-analysis of correlational studies in jamovi.
Task 2. Create a dataset for a meta-analysis of effect size differences in jamovi.

References

Borenstein, M., Hedges, L. V., Higgins, J. P. T., & Rothstein, H. R. (2005). *Comprehensive meta-analysis* (Version 2) [Computer Software]. Biostat.

Borenstein, M., Hedges, L. V., Higgins, J., & Rothstein, H. R. (2021). *Introduction to meta-analysis* (2nd ed.). Wiley.

Conner, M., Warren, R., Close, S., & Sparks, P. (1999). Alcohol consumption and the theory of planned behavior: An examination of the cognitive mediation of past behaviorid. *Journal of Applied Social Psychology, 29*(8), 1676–1704. https://doi.org/10.1111/j.1559-1816.1999.tb02046.x

Cooke, R., Dahdah, M., Norman, P., & French, D. P. (2016). How well does the theory of planned behaviour predict alcohol consumption? A systematic review and meta-analysis. *Health Psychology Review, 10*, 148–167. https://doi.org/10.1080/17437199.2014.947547

Cooke, R., McEwan, H., & Norman, P. (2023). The effect of forming implementation intentions on alcohol consumption: A systematic review and meta-analysis. *Drug and Alcohol Review, 42*, 68–80. https://doi.org/10.1111/dar.13553

Newby, K., Teah, G., Cooke, R., Li, X., Brown, K., Salisbury-Finch, B., Kwah, K., Bartle, N., Curtis, K., Fulton, E., Parsons, J., Dusseldorp, E., & Williams, S. L. (2021). Do automated digital health behaviour change interventions have a positive effect on self-efficacy? A systematic review and meta-analysis. *Health Psychology Review, 15*(1), 140–158. https://doi.org/10.1080/17437199.2019.1705873

Schwarzer, R. (1988). *Meta: Programs for secondary data analysis.* [Computer Software].
Viechtbauer, W. (2010). Conducting meta-analyses in *R* with the metafor package. *Journal of Statistical Software, 36*(3), 10.18637/jss.v036.i03.
Zimmermann, F., & Sieverding, M. (2011). Young adults' images of abstaining and drinking: Prototype dimensions, correlates and assessment methods. *Journal of Health Psychology, 16*(3), 410–420. https://doi.org/10.1177/1359105310373412

How to Conduct a Meta-Analysis of Correlations

9

Running a Meta-Analysis of Correlations in jamovi Using MAJOR

First, open jamovi and create a new file with three variables by clicking on the letters (*A*, *B*, *C*) above the dataset: Study Name; Sample Size; Correlation. Study Name is used to identify study authors/study label; it is a *nominal* measure type and *text* data type. Sample Size is the sample size for each study; it is a *continuous* measure type, and an *integer* data type. Correlation is the correlation between the variables; it is a *continuous* measure type, and a *decimal* data type. After creating the variables, enter data[1] to recreate Fig. 9.1.

You are now ready to run a meta-analysis of correlations!

Clicking on MAJOR will open a drop-down window in your dataset as in Fig. 9.2.

Select the first option—Correlation Coefficients (*r*, *N*) —to tell MAJOR you want to run a meta-analysis using correlations (*r*) and sample sizes (*N*) from a set of studies. When you click on this option, you will enter the analysis window (see Fig. 9.3) where you enter variables to run your meta-analysis of correlations.

Use the arrows in the middle of the display to match the variable names with the relevant boxes:

- Correlation➔Correlations
- Sample Size➔Sample Sizes
- Study Name➔Study Label

[1] This data is from Table 7.1 and is also available as a .csv file on my Open Science page for you to download and open in jamovi.

R. Cooke, *Meta-Analysis for Psychologists*,
https://doi.org/10.1007/978-3-031-73773-2_9

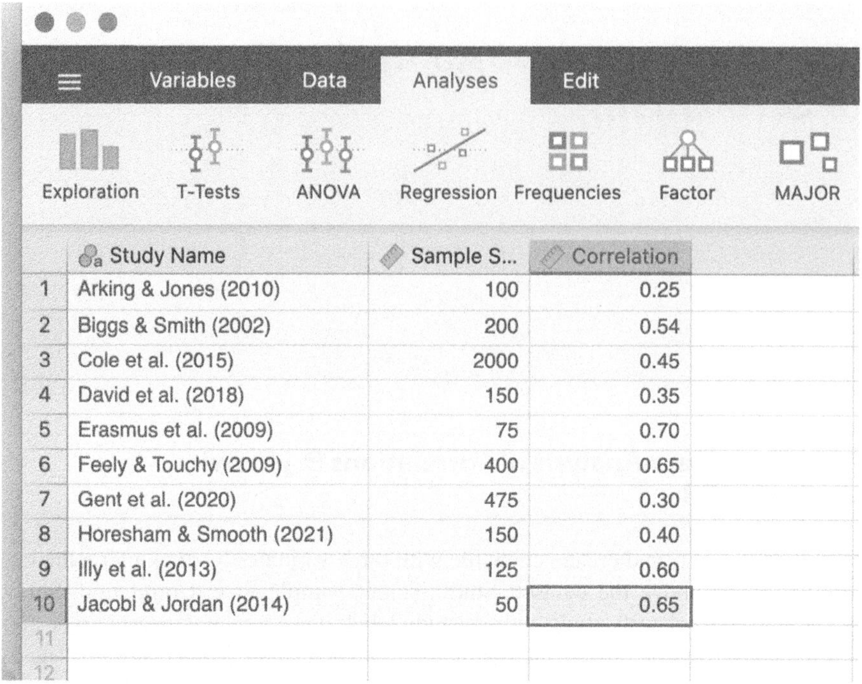

Fig. 9.1 Table 7.1 data entered into jamovi

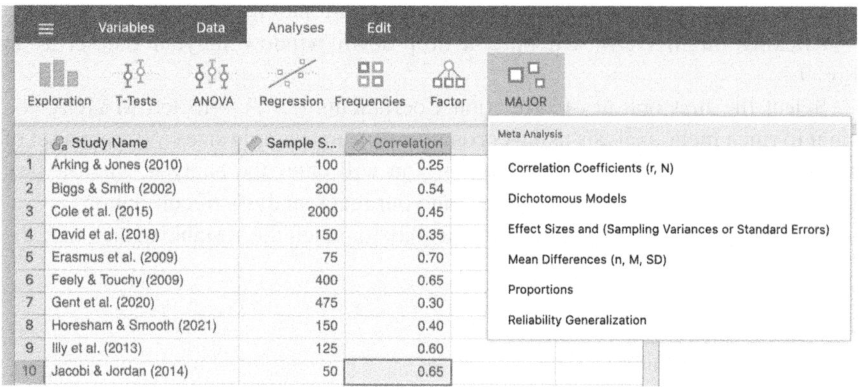

Fig. 9.2 MAJOR drop-down menu

After you do this, your output window in jamovi will populate with information about your meta-analysis. I will go slowly go through each part of this output in the next section.

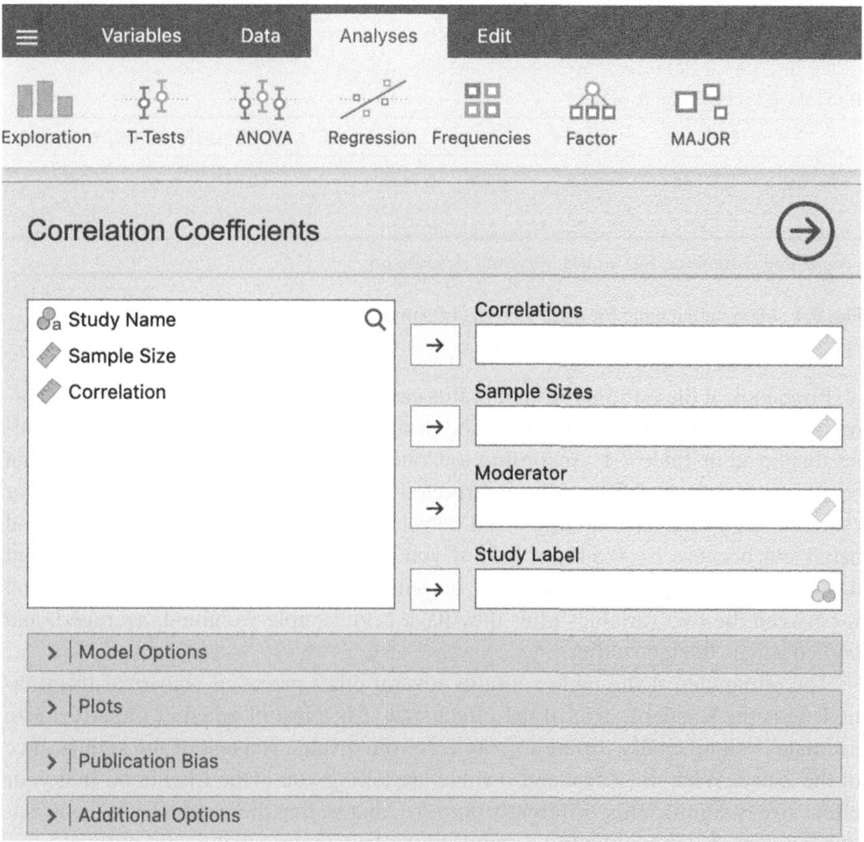

Fig. 9.3 MAJOR analysis window for correlation coefficients (*r*, *N*)

How Do I Interpret the Output?

The output is split into three sections: (1) Main output table (Fig. 9.4), which shows the overall effect size for your meta-analysis plus various statistics; (2) Tests of heterogeneity table (Fig. 9.5) and forest plot (Fig. 9.6); (3) Tests of publication bias table (Fig. 9.8) and funnel plot (Fig. 9.9). I will start by explaining the Main output table.

Main Output

The main output table contains the key statistical information from your meta-analysis. (see Fig. 9.4). The text in blue confirms the type of meta-analysis you have run in MAJOR—Correlation Coefficients using correlations and sample sizes. Immediately above the table it says a random effects model was used—I will explain this idea in Chap. 11.

Correlation Coefficients (r, N)

Random-Effects Model (k = 10)

	Estimate	se	Z	p	CI Lower Bound	CI Upper Bound
Intercept	0.546	0.0662	8.24	<.001	0.416	0.676
	.	.	.	.	.	.

Note. Tau² Estimator: Restricted Maximum-Likelihood

Fig. 9.4 Main output table for meta-analysis of correlations

First, look at the estimate, which in this case is the sample-weighted average correlation between drinking intentions and drinking behaviour, based on the ten studies displayed in Table 7.1. According to Cohen (1992), correlation coefficients that equal or exceed $r = 0.50$ can be interpreted as large-sized. Thus, we can say our estimate shows we have a large-sized correlation between drinking intentions and behaviour because $r = 0.546$, or 0.55 if you round up.[2] This is the most important information within your meta-analytic output; it tells the reader what the correlation is between the two variables after they have been sample-weighted, averaged, and pooled across the ten studies.

The remainder of the table contains several other pieces of statistical information: se is the standard error of the effect size; *Z* is a test of whether the effect size estimate is significantly different from zero; the p value is a test of the significance of the *Z* test. What the *Z* test and *p* value are telling you is the likelihood that your effect size is significantly different from zero, that is, that there actually is a correlation between drinking intentions and drinking behaviour which is not null.

Where meta-analysis differs from usual practice about reporting statistics in psychology, however, is that most of the time we're not that interested in a significant result in terms of a *p* value. Instead we use other statistics, confidence intervals, to infer significance in a meta-analysis. Because meta-analysis is about pooling results across studies, we are interested in the range of possible values the effect size estimate could take, using the data from the studies we have collected to provide this information. If your experience of statistics is focused on analysing data from a single dataset, you've probably not stopped to think about the range of values an effect size, like a correlation, could take, across a set of studies. And yet, this is a good question to ask! Every time we do a study, we are collecting data to inform ourselves about something we are interested in; in this example, the correlation between drinking intentions and drinking behaviour. A key reason to run a meta-analysis is to compare correlations from multiple studies to get a sense of the range

[2] Reporting results to two or three (or more) decimal places often generates animated arguments in statistics. I was taught to round up to two decimal places, but some journals insist on reporting three decimal places and rounding up can cause confusion and shady practice when used with p values. Tread carefully!

of values found for an effect size. Doing this helps us develop a more precise estimate of the range of values our effect size *could* take. Moving from primary to secondary analysis means thinking about the accumulation of evidence rather than the result from one study. This issue is more salient when running secondary analyses.

We have a lower limit confidence interval of 0.416, which is a medium-sized correlation, and an upper limit confidence interval of 0.676, which is a large-sized correlation. Lower and upper confidence intervals are calculated to fall above or below your effect size estimate ($r = 0.545$) and are equidistant between the lower and upper limit values. The lower value of $r = 0.416$ is 0.13 below the effect size estimate ($r = 0.545$), the upper value ($r = 0.676$) 0.13 above the estimate. So, the final thing your main table is telling you is that while the sample-weighted average correlation for your studies is $r = 0.545$, the correlation could fall anywhere between $r = 0.416$ (the lower confidence interval) and $r = 0.676$ based on data from the ten studies you included. From an interpretation point of view this means that our drinking intentions–drinking behaviour correlation is at least medium-sized (the lower value is medium-sized) and likely to be large-sized (the estimate and upper value are both large-sized).

I'll finish this section by making two additional points. First, over time, you develop an intuitive sense of wide and narrow confidence intervals. To me, these confidence intervals are narrow, meaning, that the correlation values we have across studies are similar (common with made up data!). Second, confidence intervals are easier to interpret than p values, in my opinion. To interpret an effect size estimate as significant using confidence intervals, all you need to do is check if the signs are the same: both positive or both negative means you have a significant effect. If one sign is negative and the other positive, however, that means you have a non-significant effect? Why? Because it means that *zero* is a potential value for your effect size, and if zero lies within the range of potential values for your effect size estimate, you cannot rule out the possibility that it is the 'true' effect size.

Heterogeneity Statistics

The second table in your output is titled Heterogeneity Statistics (see Fig. 9.5).

I^2 is a commonly reported measure of heterogeneity between studies included in a meta-analysis. As a heuristic, the way to interpret I^2 is if the value is below 25%, you have low heterogeneity, between 26 and 75% is moderate heterogeneity, while above 75% is high heterogeneity. In our case, the value is 91.04% indicating high heterogeneity. The Q value ($Q = 76.883$, $p < 0.001$) indicates significant heterogeneity between effect sizes included in the meta. Taken together, these statistics show that correlations between drinking intentions and behaviour vary considerably from one study to another. I'll talk about Tau and Tau^2 when I discuss differences between random effects and fixed-effect meta-analyses in Chap. 11 and provide more information on heterogeneity statistics in Chap. 12.

Heterogeneity Statistics

Tau	Tau²	I²	H²	R²	df	Q	p
0.192	0.0368 (SE= 0.0206)	91.04%	11.156	.	9.000	76.883	<.001

Fig. 9.5 Heterogeneity statistics table for meta-analysis of correlations

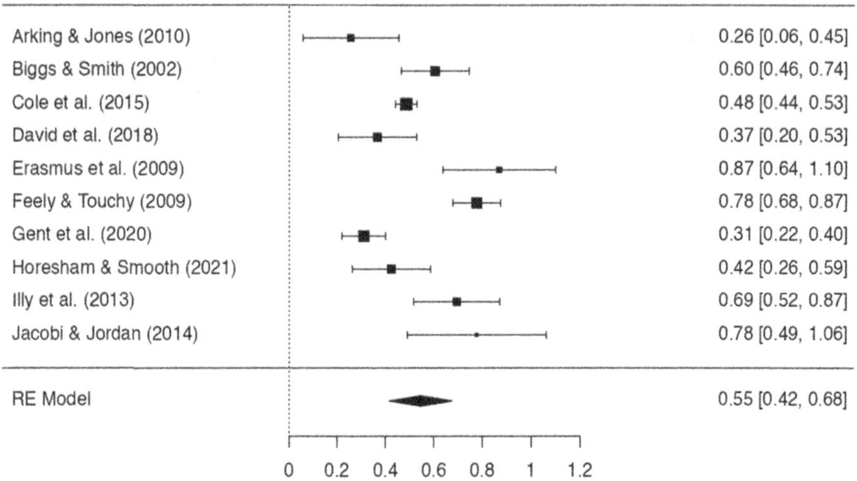

Fig. 9.6 Forest plot for meta-analysis of correlations

The forest plot (see Fig. 9.6) below the table provides a visual illustration of the heterogeneity between studies. Each square on the plot represents a correlation for one study with the arms showing the confidence intervals. There is a useful trick when it comes to inferring effects within the forest plot—the wider the confidence intervals, the smaller the sample size, and conversely, the narrower the confidence intervals, the larger the sample size. The diamond at the bottom of the plot shows the overall correlation; its edges represent the confidence intervals.

Inspecting the Forest plot you can see that correlations vary from the small-sized correlation reported by Arking and Jones (2010) $r = 0.26$ to the likely collinear large-sized correlation of $r = 0.87$ reported by Erasmus et al. (2009). Five of the studies report large-sized correlations, so we should perhaps not be too surprised that the overall effect size estimate is also large-sized.

We can add to our understanding of effect sizes included by getting MAJOR to add the weightings for each study. Remember that meta-analysis assumes that larger samples are more representative of the population effect size (see Chaps. 3 and 7), which means that of these ten studies, Cole et al. should be more representative of the population effect size than Jacobi and Jordan. We can confirm our reasoning by using one of the menus in jamovi. If you click on the plots menu, you can add the Model fitting weights to the forest plot. These weights tell you how much each study informs the overall effect size.

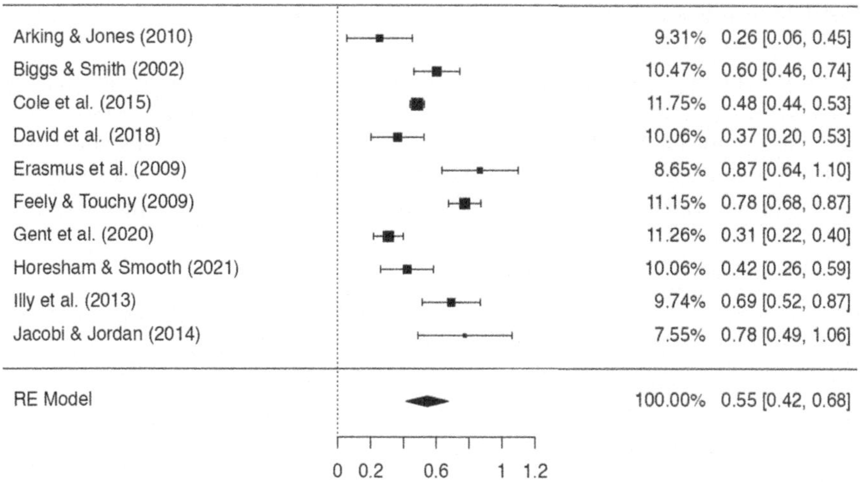

Fig. 9.7 Forest plot with study weightings added

Confirming our belief in the importance of Cole et al., we can see in Fig. 9.7 that this study had 11.75% weight (influence) on the overall effect size. As mentioned above, Jacobi and Jordan (2014) has the lowest weight (influence) 7.55%, due to having the smallest sample size of our studies. The takeaway message from this digression is that the overall correlation depends more on correlations from larger samples than correlations from smaller samples. This is the genius of meta-analysis; Jacobi and Jordan's (2014) large correlation ($r = 0.78$) is unlikely to be the population correlation between drinking intentions and behaviour because it is based on a small sample size, which are prone to being unreliable. In contrast, a correlation from a larger sample, like Cole et al.'s (2015) $r = 0.48$ is more likely to reflect the population correlation and is a better basis for inference. I will discuss weighting studies in more detail in Chap. 11.

There are a couple of other things you can infer from this forest plot. Each study has an effect size difference to the right of the vertical line, which is set at zero meaning no correlation between intentions and behaviour. So, all our included studies reported positive correlations.

As well as checking the direction of each study from the forest plot, we can also check the magnitude of the effect size for each study. Taking this idea a step further, the forest plot allows us to identify any effect sizes that are not significantly different from zero, by examining the confidence intervals for each study. In this set of studies, none of the confidence intervals contain zero, meaning that all results are significant. This does not mean all included studies show a 'true' effect, however. It is possible that some results reflect p-hacking (see Chap. 13). This leads us neatly on to discuss the table showing Publication Bias Assessment statistics.

Publication Bias

The final table in your output provides information about publication bias, that is, the tendency for journals to publish papers reporting significant findings (see Chap. 13), like significant correlations between variables. Two methods—statistical estimates of publication (see Fig. 9.8) and funnel plots (see Fig. 9.9)—are reported following meta-analyses to help identify publication bias in research literatures.

Publication Bias Assessment

Test Name	value	p
Fail-Safe N	2644.000	<.001
Begg and Mazumdar Rank Correlation	0.180	0.472
Egger's Regression	0.974	0.330
Trim and Fill Number of Studies	0.000	.

Note. Fail-safe N Calculation Using the Rosenthal Approach

Fig. 9.8 Publication bias assessment table for meta-analysis of correlations

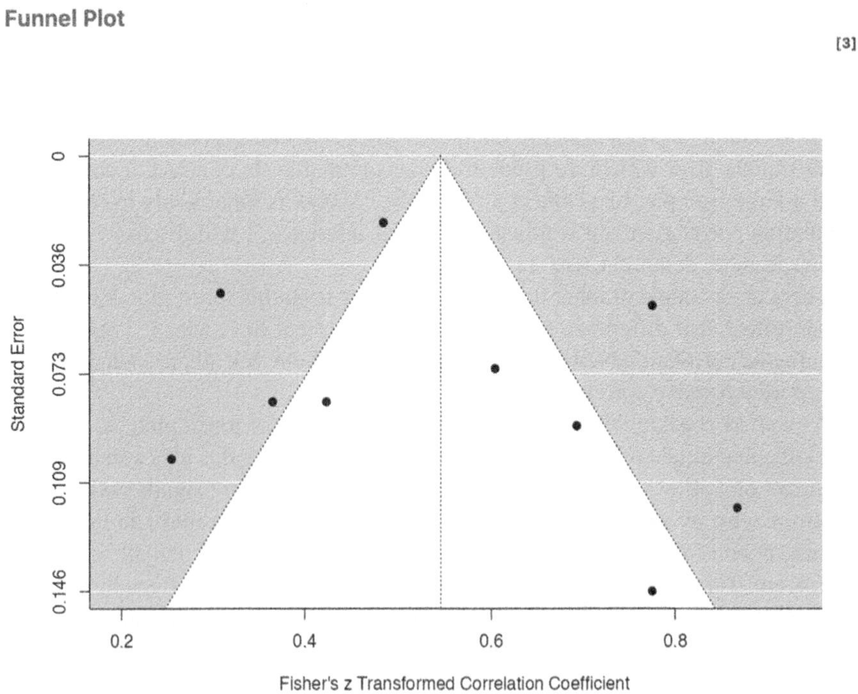

Fig. 9.9 Funnel plot for meta-analysis of correlations

Statistical Estimates of Publication Bias

Rosenthal's (1979) Fail-Safe *N* statistic tells you how many studies you would need to find that **all** show null effect sizes (correlations in this case) to reduce confidence in your meta-analytic results. You contrast Fail-Safe *N* values with the number of studies included in your meta-analysis. In this case, you have found ten studies and the fail-safe *n* value = 2644 studies. Given you spent ages systematically searching and screening and found ten studies, it seems highly unlikely that you have missed an additional 2644 studies that **ALL** report null correlations!!! So, we can infer confidence in our correlation from fail-safe values.

Begg and Mazumdar's (1994) Rank Correlation and Egger's Test (1997) regression test both estimate the extent of symmetry in effect sizes from included studies. In a symmetrical distribution of effect sizes, you should have a roughly equal number of effects above and below the overall estimate. This would indicate that studies with smaller, null, or negative effects, which are less likely to be significant, are being published. In an asymmetrical distribution, in contrast, studies reporting smaller, null, or negative effects, which are less likely to be significant, are missing from the plot. Hence, there is a lack of symmetry in the distribution of effect sizes.

An additional indicator of publication bias is when your set of studies ONLY include studies with small sample sizes reporting positive and significant effect sizes and lacks studies with small sample sizes with negative (or null) effect sizes. Assuming publication bias exists, the studies with significant effects are more likely to be published than the studies with non-significant effect sizes, even if these studies, when based on small sample sizes, might produce unreliable effects. In our table, both statistics are not significant which suggests an absence of publication bias. We can also look at a funnel plot to check for publication bias.

Funnel Plot as a Visual Indicator of Publication Bias

Interpreting a funnel plot (Fig. 9.9) centres on thinking about included studies' effects in terms of their magnitude and standard errors, which are an analogue of sample size. Effect sizes (correlations here) are plotted on the *X* axis. For instance, at the bottom of the plot nearest the *X* axis, Jacobi and Jordan's r of 0.78; near the top of the plot, to the left of the vertical line, you can see Cole et al. $r = 0.48$. The effect sizes are spread apart in this plot because they vary in sample size, and therefore, sample error, which is plotted on the *Y* axis.

As discussed in Chap. 7, studies with larger sample sizes necessarily possess smaller standard errors relative to studies with smaller sample sizes. Standard errors represent the distance between an individual effect size from the overall (population) effect size, for example, the distance between Cole et al.'s $r = 0.48$ and the overall effect size $r = 0.55$, adjusted by the sample size for the individual effect size. The reason that Jacobi and Jordan has a larger standard error than Cole et al. is that it has a smaller sample size. We can use our forest plot to identify effect sizes and then use the funnel plot to identify which studies have the smallest standard errors.

Small and large are both relative terms here; a small standard error in this Funnel plot might be a large standard error in another sample of studies.

Although you can use the funnel plot to check results for individual studies, most of the time we use them to visualize the distribution of effect sizes and see if they appear symmetrical or asymmetrical; asymmetrical effect sizes suggest publication bias. Figure 9.9 shows a symmetrical distribution: five effect sizes appear to the right of the population estimate ($r = 0.55$) and five appear to the left of it. While there are no studies to the left of the vertical line, indicating studies reporting smaller correlation that also have a large standard error, there is only Jacobi and Jordan's paper that is to the right of the vertical line with a large standard error; this is the kind of result that suggests an unreliable finding, perhaps even evidence of *p*-hacking. In a literature where publication bias is present, you would expect there to be more studies in this sector of the plot.

While you cannot rule out publication bias based on the symmetry of a funnel plot (Borenstein et al., 2021), the non-significance of Begg and Mazumdar's Rank Correlation (1994) and Egger's Test (1997) regression statistics reported in the table increases confidence that our set of studies is not too badly affected by publication bias. Interpreting results from meta-analysis often involves constructing arguments based on multiple sources of information. If the funnel plot looks symmetrical and the statistics are non-significant, you can propose a lack of publication bias. Conversely, an asymmetrical distribution and significant statistics suggests your set of included studies may suffer from publication bias. I will pick up these issues in greater depth in Chap. 13.

Summary

You now know how to run a meta-analysis of correlations in jamovi using MAJOR and how to interpret the output. When writing up the results of your meta-analysis, always report the overall effect size, confidence intervals, tests of heterogeneity, and publication bias in the main text and include relevant forest plot(s) as a figure(s) (see Chap. 15 for more tips on how to write-up your results). You can include a funnel plot(s) too, but I usually include them as supplementary files, especially if they show symmetry. To help reinforce your learning of the material covered in this chapter, I've included some tasks to help you practise your skills.

Tasks

Task 1: Report the key information from the main output table of your meta-analysis.

Task 2: Report the heterogeneity of your meta-analysis.

Task 3: Report the evidence for/against publication bias in your meta-analysis.

Task 4: Go back to your dataset and change the sample sizes of these studies as follows:

- Cole et al. (2015) change from $N = 2000$ to $N = 200$
- Jacobi and Jordan (2014) change from $N = 75$ to $N = 750$

Then re-run your meta-analysis. Compare the results to your answers for Tasks 1–3 and see if any changes have taken place that affect your interpretation of the results.

Task 5: Copy your original dataset (give it the name: 'Eight correlations'). Remove Jacobi and Jordan and Erasmus et al. and see what impact that has on (1) the main output table, (2) the heterogeneity table, and most critically (3) the funnel plot.

References

Begg, C. B., & Mazumdar, M. (1994). Operating characteristics of a rank correlation test for publication bias. *Biometrics, 50*, 1088–1101.

Borenstein, M., Hedges, L. V., Higgins, J., & Rothstein, H. R. (2021). *Introduction to meta-analysis (Second edition)*. Wiley.

Cohen, J. (1992). A power primer. *Psychological Bulletin, 112*(1), 155–159.

Egger, M., Higgins, J. P. T., & Smith, D. (1997). Bias in meta-analysis detected by a simple, graphical test. *BMJ, 315*, 629–634.

Rosenthal, R. R. (1979). The File drawer problem and tolerance for null results. *Psychological Bulletin, 86*, 638–641.

How to Conduct a Meta-Analysis of Effect Size Differences

10

Running a Meta-Analysis of Effect Size Differences in Jamovi Using MAJOR

In Chap. 8, I contrasted two methods of creating a dataset for meta-analyses of effect size differences: Method (1), where you enter the mean, standard deviation, and sample size for each group (control, experiment/intervention) and Method (2), where you enter the calculated effect size differences and the sample error/study variance. As noted in Chap. 8, I prefer method (1) when conducting meta-analyses of effect size differences because it saves me the effort of calculating effect size differences and generating the sample error/study variance. So, I'm going to explain how to use method (1) in this chapter. We will use data displayed in Table 10.1, an expanded version of Table 7.2, containing raw statistics.

Get started by opening a new jamovi file and creating the following seven variables:

1. Study Name (to identify the study authors, a nominal measure, and text data type)
2. Control N (the sample size for the control group/condition; a continuous measure and integer data type)
3. Control M (the mean for the outcome in the control group; a continuous measure and usually a decimal data type)
4. Control SD (the standard deviation for the outcome in the control group; a continuous measure and usually a decimal data type)
5. Experiment N (the sample size for the experimental or intervention group/condition; a continuous measure and integer data type)
6. Experiment M (the mean for the outcome in the experimental or intervention group; a continuous measure and usually a decimal data type)
7. Experiment SD (the standard deviation for the outcome in the experimental or intervention group; a continuous measure and usually a decimal data type)

R. Cooke, *Meta-Analysis for Psychologists*,
https://doi.org/10.1007/978-3-031-73773-2_10

Table 10.1 Raw statistics for studies testing interventions to reduce screen time

Authors	Control			Intervention		
	M	SD	N	M	SD	N
Keane et al.	13.50	4.90	50	12.50	4.88	50
Linus et al.	10.00	2.20	75	8.75	1.99	75
Mimms et al.	15.00	4.00	25	12.00	4.40	25
Noone et al.	20.00	5.15	125	17.00	4.20	120
Owen	17.00	3.12	250	13.5	6.10	200
Peeps et al.	14.00	7.88	500	11.50	4.30	450
Quest et al.	25.00	4.50	15	24.00	4.30	20
Ricki et al.	13.00	2.20	115	11.50	3.90	120
Sopp et al.	18.00	3.50	55	15.50	7.50	45
Tapp et al.	30.00	4.00	30	27.00	3.50	20

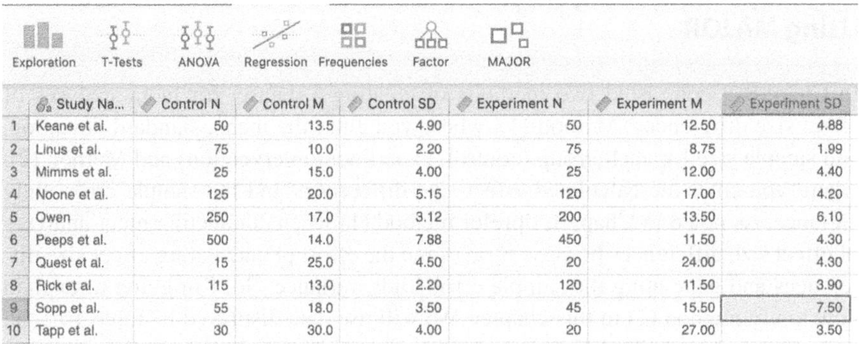

	Study Na...	Control N	Control M	Control SD	Experiment N	Experiment M	Experiment SD
1	Keane et al.	50	13.5	4.90	50	12.50	4.88
2	Linus et al.	75	10.0	2.20	75	8.75	1.99
3	Mimms et al.	25	15.0	4.00	25	12.00	4.40
4	Noone et al.	125	20.0	5.15	120	17.00	4.20
5	Owen	250	17.0	3.12	200	13.50	6.10
6	Peeps et al.	500	14.0	7.88	450	11.50	4.30
7	Quest et al.	15	25.0	4.50	20	24.00	4.30
8	Rick et al.	115	13.0	2.20	120	11.50	3.90
9	Sopp et al.	55	18.0	3.50	45	15.50	7.50
10	Tapp et al.	30	30.0	4.00	20	27.00	3.50

Fig. 10.1 Data from Table 7.2 entered into jamovi

Next enter the data[1] from Table 10.1, to recreate Fig. 10.1.

You are now ready to run a meta-analysis of effect size differences!

Clicking on MAJOR will open a drop-down menu in your dataset, as in Fig. 10.2. Select the fourth option—Mean Differences (n, M, SD) —to tell MAJOR you want to run a meta-analysis of effect size differences using sample size (n), mean (M), and standard deviation (SD) for the two groups. When you click on this option, you will enter the analysis window (see Fig. 10.3) where you enter variables to run your meta-analysis of effect size differences.

Use the arrows in the middle of the display to match the variables with the relevant boxes:

- Group One Sample Size→Control N
- Group One Mean→Control M
- Group One Standard Deviation→Control SD

[1] This data is also available on my Open Science Framework page as a csv file you can download and open in jamovi.

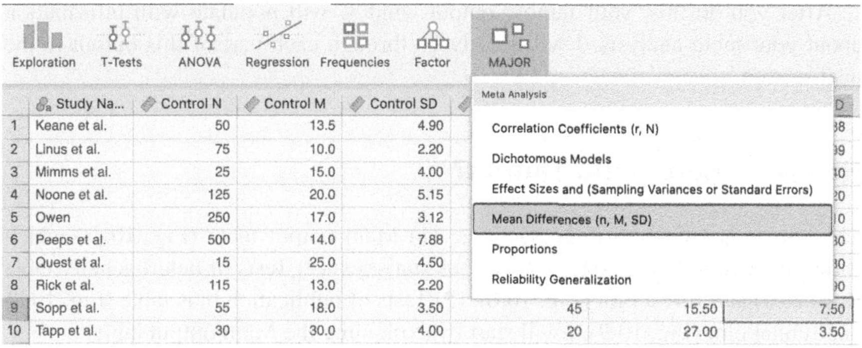

Fig. 10.2 MAJOR drop-down menu

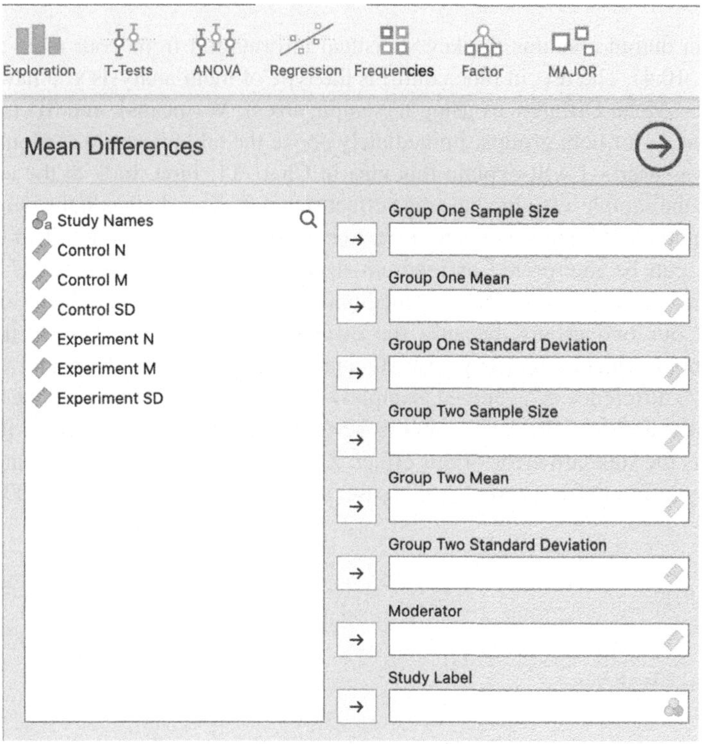

Fig. 10.3 MAJOR analysis window for Mean Differences (n, M, SD)

- Group Two Sample Size→Experiment N
- Group Two Mean→Experiment M
- Group Two Standard Deviation→Experiment SD
- Study Label→Study Names

After you do this, your jamovi output window will populate with information about your meta-analysis. I will slowly go through each part of this output in the next section.

How Do I Interpret the Output?

The output is split into three sections: (1) Main output table (Fig. 10.4), which shows the overall effect size plus various statistics; (2) Tests of heterogeneity table (Fig. 10.5) and forest plot (Fig. 10.6); (3) Tests of publication bias table (Fig. 10.8) and funnel plot (Fig. 10.9). I will start by explaining the Main output table.

Main Output

The main output contains the key statistical information from your meta-analysis (see Fig. 10.4). The text in blue confirms the type of meta-analysis you have run in MAJOR—Mean Differences using n (sample sizes), M (means), and SD (standard deviations)—for both groups. Immediately above the table it says a random effects model was used—I will explain this idea in Chap. 11. First, look at the estimate, which is the sample-weighted average effect size difference between the two groups in the outcome of interest (screen time). According to Cohen (1992), effect size differences can be interpreted as medium-sized if they equal or exceed d = 0.50. Therefore, we can say we have a medium effect size difference in the outcome between our two groups because the estimate is d = 0.524. This is the most important information within your meta-analytic output; it tells the reader what the effect size difference is, averaged, sample-weighted, and pooled across the studies.

The remainder of the table contains several other pieces of statistical information: se is the standard error of this effect; Z is a test of whether the estimate is significantly different from zero—in this case, it is because the p value is <0.001. What

Results

Meta-Analysis

Random-Effects Model (k = 10)

	Estimate	se	Z	p	CI Lower Bound	CI Upper Bound
Intercept	0.524	0.0633	8.28	<.001	0.400	0.648

Note. Tau² Estimator: Restricted Maximum-Likelihood

[3]

Fig. 10.4 Main output table for meta-analysis of effect size differences

the Z test and *p* value are telling you is the likelihood that your effect size is significantly different from zero; put another way, that there actually is an effect size difference in screen time between control and intervention groups and it is not null.

Now a key difference with reporting meta-analysis is that the preference is to focus on the confidence intervals, in this case 0.400 and 0.648, rather than Z and *p* values. Meta-analyses tend to focus on the confidence intervals, instead of the Z and *p* values, because it helps with inferences about the range of values reported across studies, an issue that is more salient when running secondary analyses. We have a lower limit confidence interval of 0.400, which is a small effect size difference, and an upper limit confidence interval of 0.648, which is a medium effect size difference. Your overall effect will always fall equidistant between the lower and upper limit values; it is 0.124 above the lower limit value and 0.124 below it. Overall, the values tell us that the effect of receiving an intervention to reduce screen time in the included studies produced somewhere between a small-sized and medium-sized effect size difference in screen time.

I'll finish this section by making two additional points. First, over time, you develop an intuitive sense of wide and narrow confidence intervals. To me, these confidence intervals are narrow meaning that the effect size difference values we have across studies are like one another (common with made up data!). Second, confidence intervals are easier to interpret in terms of significance, than *p* values. To interpret an effect as significant using confidence intervals, all you need to do is check if the signs are the same: both positive or both negative means you have a significant effect. If one sign is negative and the other positive, however, that means you have a non-significant effect? Why? Because it means that the value zero is a potential value for your effect, and if zero is a potential value you cannot rule out the possibility that it is the 'true' effect size.

Heterogeneity Statistics

The second table in your output is titled Heterogeneity Statistics (see Fig. 10.5). I^2 is a commonly reported measure of heterogeneity between studies included in a meta-analysis. As a heuristic, the way to interpret I^2 is if the value is below 25%, you have low heterogeneity, between 26 and 75% is moderate heterogeneity, while above 75% is high heterogeneity. In our case the value is 40.25% indicating moderate heterogeneity. The Q value is non-significant (Q = 14.883, p = 0.094) which suggests a lack of heterogeneity in effect sizes between studies. Taken together, these statistics show that while effect size differences vary from one study to another,

Heterogeneity Statistics

Tau	Tau²	I²	H²	R²	df	Q	p
0.118	0.0139 (SE= 0.0171)	40.25%	1.674	.	9.000	14.883	0.094

Fig. 10.5 Heterogeneity statistics table for meta-analysis of effect size differences

Forest Plot

[3]

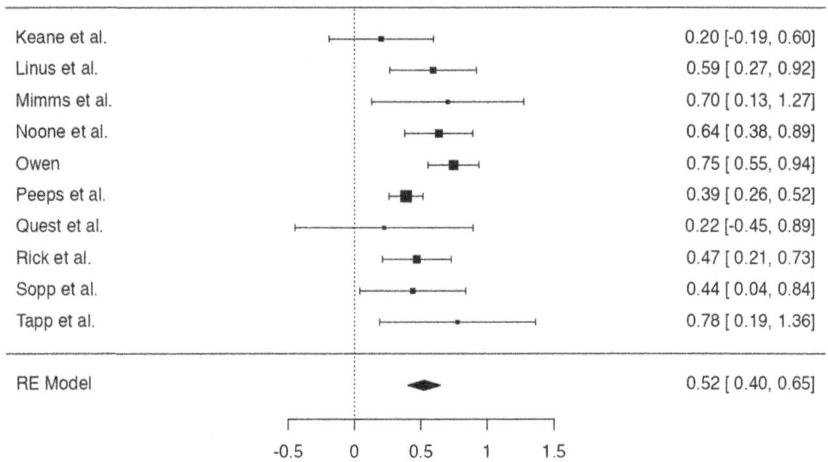

Fig. 10.6 Forest plot for meta-analysis of effect size differences

this variance is not particularly large. I'll talk about Tau and Tau^2 when I discuss differences between random effects and fixed effect meta-analyses in Chap. 11 and go into the heterogeneity statistics in more detail in Chap. 12.

The forest plot (Fig. 10.6) provides a visualisation of the effect sizes from included studies and confirms that the effect size differences do not vary much between studies. Each square on the plot represents an effect size difference for one study with the arms showing the confidence intervals. There is a useful trick when it comes to inferring effects within the forest plot—the wider the confidence intervals, the smaller the sample size, and conversely, the narrower the confidence intervals the larger the sample size. The diamond at the bottom of the plot shows the overall effect size difference; its edges represent the confidence intervals.

Based on this forest plot, most effect size differences are similar. Sopp et al. ($d = 0.44$); Rick et al. ($d = 0.47$); Linus et al. ($d = 0.59$) and Noone et al. ($d = 0.64$) all fall within the overall confidence intervals of [0.40; 0.65] with Peeps et al. ($d = 0.39$) just below the lower interval. The other five studies are more variable: Keane et al. ($d = 0.20$) and Quest et al. ($d = 0.22$) are both small-sized; Mimms et al. ($d = 0.70$), Owen ($d = 0.75$) and Tapp et al. ($d = 0.78$) are all medium-sized. So, our range of effect size differences is from $d = 0.20$ (Keane et al.) to $d = 0.78$ (Tapp et al.). While this is quite a wide range of values, the fact that four studies lie within the confidence intervals, with one close to the lower limit, shows there is some degree of replication of effect sizes in these included studies. The studies are not all finding completely different things, which is an encouraging sign as the goal of meta-analysis is to provide a precise effect size from studies reporting on the same phenomenon.

We can add to our understanding of effect sizes for included studies by getting MAJOR to add the weightings for each study. Remember that meta-analysis assumes that larger samples are more representative of the population effect size (see Chaps. 3 and 7), which means that of these ten studies, Peeps et al. should be more representative of the population effect size than Quest et al. We can confirm our reasoning by using one of the menus in jamovi. If you click on the plots menu, you can add the Model fitting weights to the Forest plot. These weights tell you how much each study informs the overall effect size and are shown in Fig. 10.7. We can see from this image that Peeps et al. had 22.04% weight (influence) on the overall effect size. In contrast, Quest et al. had only 3.05% weighting and Tapp et al. 3.88% weighting; their small sample sizes counted against them.

The takeaway message is that the overall effect size difference depends more on effect size differences from larger samples than effect size differences from smaller samples. This is important when evaluating interventions—showing a significant effect size difference for an intervention based on a smaller sample size can lead to overconfidence, showing a significant effect size difference for an intervention with a larger sample size gives you much greater confidence in your findings. Pooling results gives you the greatest confidence of all because you are moving away

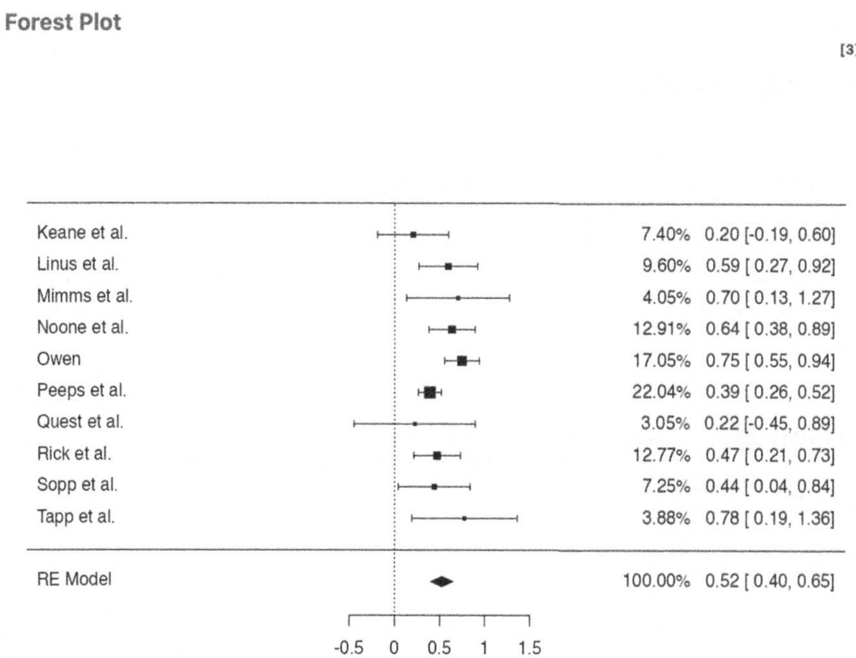

Fig. 10.7 Forest plot with study weightings added

interpreting effects of an intervention based on one set of results, or a handful of results, to a position where you are synthesising all available data to give you a range of possible values.

There's a couple of other things you can infer from this forest plot. Each study has an effect size difference to the right of the vertical line, which is set at zero meaning no difference in the outcome between the two groups. So, all our included studies reported results that favoured the intervention over control, that is, screen time reduced more in the intervention group than the control group at follow-up (see Chap. 7 for more on this point).

As well as checking the direction of each study from the forest plot, we can also check the magnitude of the effect size for each study. Taking this idea a step further, the forest plot allows us to identify effect sizes that are not significantly different from zero, by examining the confidence intervals for each study. Looking at Fig. 10.7, you will see two studies that have effect size differences that are not significantly different from zero: Quest et al. has a lower confidence interval of $d = -0.45$, to go with an upper confidence interval of $d = 0.89$; Keane et al. has a lower confidence interval of $d = -0.19$ and an upper confidence interval of $d = 0.60$. As noted above, when your confidence intervals contain one negative and one positive value that means they also contain zero as a possible value, which means they are not significantly different from zero. In both cases, the studies have small sample sizes for each group. Quest et al. had 15 control participants and 20 intervention participants. Keane et al. had 50 in each group. Small sample sizes beget wide confidence intervals. Something to watch out for in your meta-analysis…

Publication Bias

The final table in your output provides information about publication bias, that is, the tendency for journals to publish papers reporting significant findings, like significant effect size differences that favour the intervention group over the control (see Chap. 13).

Two methods—statistical estimates of publication (see Fig. 10.8) and funnel plots (see Fig. 10.9)—are reported following meta-analyses to help identify publication bias.

Statistical Estimates of Publication Bias

Rosenthal's (1979) Fail-Safe N statistic tells you how many studies you would need to find that all show null effect sizes (effect size differences in this case) to reduce confidence in your meta-analytic results. You contrast Fail-Safe N values with the number of studies included in your meta-analysis. In this case, you have found ten studies and the fail-safe n value = 425. Given you spent ages systematically searching your literature and found ten studies, it seems highly unlikely that you have missed an additional 425 studies that **ALL** report null effect size differences!!! So,

Publication Bias Assessment

Test Name	value	p
Fail-Safe N	425.000	<.001
Begg and Mazumdar Rank Correlation	−0.067	0.862
Egger's Regression	−0.086	0.931
Trim and Fill Number of Studies	0.000	.

Note. Fail-safe N Calculation Using the Rosenthal Approach

Fig. 10.8 Publication Bias Assessment table for meta-analysis of effect size differences

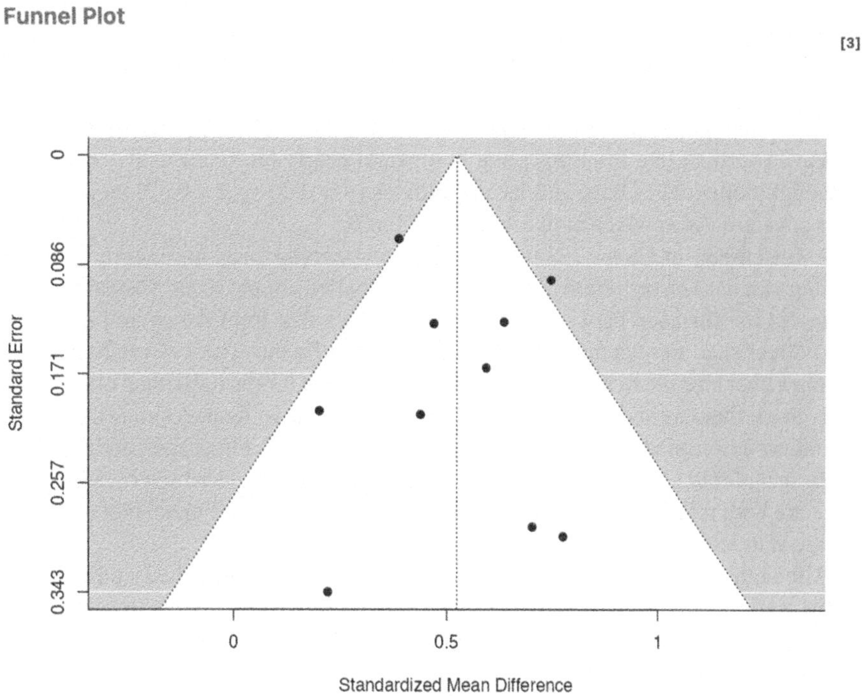

Fig. 10.9 Funnel plot for meta-analysis of effect size differences

we can infer confidence in our correlation from this statistic by reporting the Fail-Safe N value.

Begg and Mazumdar's (1994) Rank Correlation and Egger's Test (1997) regression test both estimate the extent of symmetry in effect sizes from included studies. In a symmetrical distribution of effect sizes you should have a roughly equal number of effects above and below the overall estimate. This would indicate that studies with smaller, null, or negative effects that are less likely to be significant are being published. In an asymmetrical distribution, in contrast, studies reporting smaller, null, or negative effects, that are less likely to be significant, are missing from the plot. Hence, there is a lack of symmetry in the distribution of effect sizes. An additional indicator of publication bias is when your set of studies ONLY include studies with small sample sizes reporting positive and significant effect sizes and lacks studies with small sample sizes with negative (or null) effect sizes. Assuming publication bias exists, the studies with positive effects are more likely to be published than the studies with negative effect sizes, even if these studies, when based on small sample sizes, might produce unreliable effects. In our table, both statistics are non-significant suggesting a lack of publication bias.

Funnel Plot as a Visual Indicator of Publication Bias

Interpreting a funnel plot (see Fig. 10.9) centres on thinking about included studies' effects in terms of their magnitude and standard errors, which are an analogue of sample size. Effect size differences are plotted on the X axis. For instance, at the bottom of the plot nearest the X axis, you'll find Quest et al.'s *d* of 0.22. If you were to draw a vertical line from this point you would nearly hit Keane et al.'s $d = 0.20$. Although both studies have similar magnitudes ($d = 0.20$ vs $d = 0.22$) they vary in their standard error, which is plotted on the Y axis.

As discussed in Chap. 7, studies with larger sample sizes necessarily possess smaller standard errors relative to studies with smaller sample sizes. Standard errors represent the distance between an individual effect size from the overall (population) effect size, for example, the distance between Keane et al.'s $d = 0.20$ and the overall effect size $d = 0.52$, adjusted by the sample size for the individual effect size. The reason that Quest et al. has a larger standard error than Keane et al. is that it has a smaller sample size. We can use our forest plot to identify effect sizes and then use the funnel plot to identify which studies have the smallest standard errors. Small and large are both relative terms here; a small standard error in this Funnel plot might be a large standard error in another sample of studies.

Although you can use the funnel plot to check results for individual studies, most of the time we use them to visualize the distribution of effect sizes to see if they appear symmetrical or asymmetrical; asymmetrical effect sizes suggest publication bias. Fig. 10.9 shows a symmetrical distribution: five effect sizes appear to the right of the population estimate ($d = 0.52$) and five appear to the left of it. Importantly, there is one study to the left of the population estimate that also has a large standard error. This is the type of study we would expect to fall foul of publication bias so the fact we've found it encourages us that our set of included studies does not suffer from publication bias.

While you cannot rule out publication bias based on the symmetry of a Funnel plot (Borenstein et al., 2021), the non-significance of Begg and Mazumdar's (1994) Rank Correlation and Egger's Test (1997) regression statistics reported in the table increases confidence that our set of studies is not too badly affected by publication bias. Interpreting results from meta-analysis often involves constructing arguments based on multiple sources of information. If the funnel plot looks symmetrical and the statistics are non-significant, you can propose a lack of publication bias.

Conversely, an asymmetrical distribution and significant statistics suggests your set of included studies may suffer from publication bias. We'll pick up these issues in greater depth in Chap. 13.

Summary

You now know how to run a meta-analysis of effect size differences in jamovi using MAJOR and how to interpret the output. When writing up the results of your meta-analysis, always report the overall effect size, confidence intervals, tests of heterogeneity, and publication bias in the main text and include relevant forest plot(s) as a figure(s) (see Chap. 15 for more tips on how to write-up your results). You can include a funnel plot(s) too, but I usually include them as supplementary files, especially if they show symmetry. In the next chapter, we'll discuss a key conceptual issue—the difference between Random effects and Fixed-effect meta-analytic methods.

Tasks

Task 1: Report the key information from the main output table of your meta-analysis.

Task 2: Report the heterogeneity of your meta-analysis.

Task 3: Report evidence for/against publication bias in your meta-analysis.

Task 4: Go back to your dataset and change the sample sizes of these studies as follows:

- Cole et al. (2015) change from $N = 2000$ to $N = 200$
- Jacobi and Jordan (2014) change from $N = 75$ to $N = 750$

Then re-run your meta-analysis. Compare the results to your answers for Tasks 1–3 and see if any changes have taken place that affect your interpretation of the results.

Task 5: Copy your original jamovi dataset (give it the name: 'Eight effect size differences'). Remove Keane et al. and Quest et al. and see what impact that has on (1) the main output table, (2) the heterogeneity table, and most critically (3) the funnel plot.

References

Begg, C. B., & Mazumdar, M. (1994). Operating characteristics of a rank correlation test for publication bias. *Biometrics, 50*, 1088–1101.

Borenstein, M., Hedges, L. V., Higgins, J., & Rothstein, H. R. (2021). *Introduction to meta-analysis* (2nd ed.). Wiley.

Cohen, J. (1992). A power primer. *Psychological Bulletin, 112*(1), 155–159.

Egger, M., Higgins, J. P. T., & Smith, D. (1997). Bias in meta-analysis detected by a simple, graphical test. *BMJ, 315*, 629–634.

Rosenthal, R. R. (1979). The File drawer problem and tolerance for null results. *Psychological Bulletin, 86*, 638–641.

Part IV

Further Issues in Meta-Analysis

Fixed Effect vs Random Effects Meta-Analyses

11

What Kind of Meta-Analysis Should I Run?

There's a lot of information to take on board when learning about meta-analysis so I decided to focus in Part III on the nuts and bolts of running and interpreting meta-analyses, rather than discuss a key conceptual issue—what kind of meta-analysis should I run? It's now time to take a step back to think about how meta-analysis works, answering questions like "How are the included studies weighted?" and "Why are they weighted as they are?" Doing this will help you understand meta-analytic results in greater depth and help you to justify the approach you have taken. Like any statistical test, there are differences of opinion about the best way to run analyses, so, you need to know about fixed effect and random effects meta-analysis to know how to argue your case. This is important when writing up your meta-analysis (see Chap. 15).

What Kinds of Meta-Analysis Are There?

There are two kinds of meta-analysis: Fixed-effect and Random effects. In a Fixed-effect meta-analysis, it is assumed there is one 'true' (Fixed) effect size, whereas in a random effects meta-analysis, it is assumed there are a range of 'true' effect sizes that vary between studies. MAJOR's default is to run a random effects model, using the Restricted Maximum-Likelihood method although you can choose between models by clicking on the Model estimator drop-down menu (see Fig. 11.1). I have used the Hunter-Schmidt method (Cooke & French, 2008; Cooke & Sheeran, 2004) DerSimonian and Laird method (Cooke et al., 2016), or the Restricted Maximum-Likelihood method (Cooke et al., 2023), which are all random effects methods. Differences between these methods are discussed in Borenstein et al. (2021). I'm going to explain fixed-effect meta-analysis first as it is simpler to understand.

R. Cooke, *Meta-Analysis for Psychologists*,
https://doi.org/10.1007/978-3-031-73773-2_11

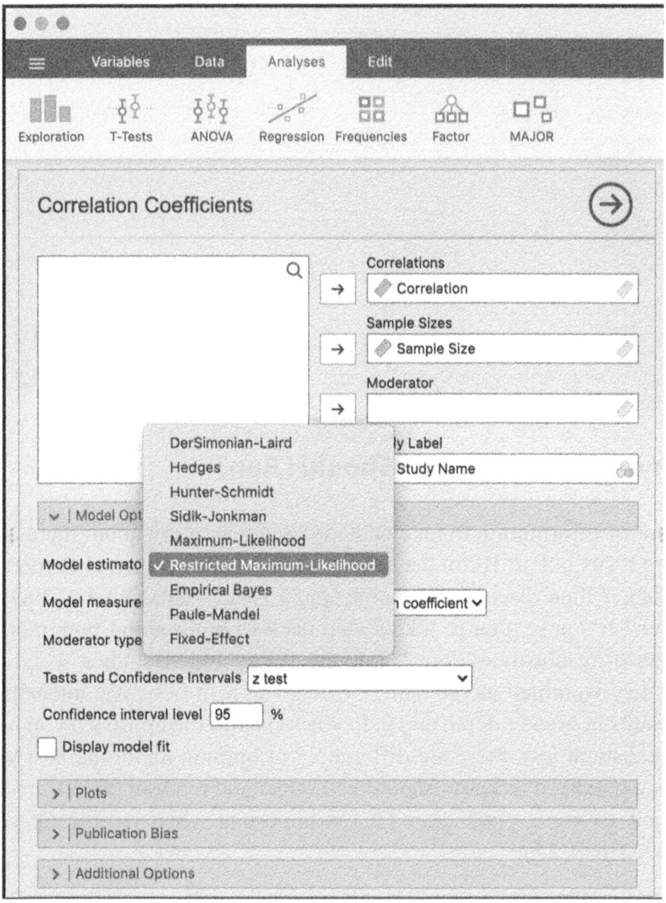

Fig. 11.1 Model estimator options

What Is a Fixed Effect Meta-Analysis?

A fixed-effect meta-analysis operates under the assumption that there is a 'true' (Fixed) effect size common to all studies that test the effect size you are interested in, like the correlation between drinking intentions and drinking behaviour, or the effect size difference in screen time between intervention and control group participants. If each study was to recruit a large enough sample drawn from the same population, using equivalent measures, et cetera, they should return the same effect size. Of course, most studies don't recruit large enough samples and, as a result, their statistics contain sampling error, which means the effect observed in each study is not the same as the true effect. This means if we want to estimate the overall effect size, we need to account for sampling error, which we estimate by using the variance of each study. Smaller samples have higher variance than larger samples,

Table 11.1 Variances and weightings for five studies

Study	Variance	Weighting (1/variance)
Kubrick	0.002	500
Kurosawa	0.004	250
Renoir	0.059	16.94
Scorsese	0.010	100
Welles	0.021	47.62

which means they also have larger sampling errors. Therefore, a fixed-effect meta-analysis assigns greater weight to studies with larger samples as they contain lower sampling error. The formula for working out the weighting of each study in a fixed-effect meta is the inverse of the variance (i.e. 1/variance); because studies with larger samples have smaller variance, they are given more weight. Table 11.1 contains the variance and weightings for five studies.

In this set of studies, Kubrick has the lowest variance, so they end up with the highest weighting. In the meta-analysis, these (absolute) values are adjusted to provide a relative weighting, where all the values add up to 100%. So, a fixed-effect meta-analysis is quite straightforward: We assume that all studies are providing a test of a true (Fixed) effect size, and we use that assumption to justify the weighting of each study being solely based on sample size when we pool results. Things are more complex in a random-effects meta-analysis.

How Does Random Effects Meta-Analysis Differ from Fixed Effect Meta-Analysis?

Random effects meta-analysis assumes that sample size is not the only source of variance between studies included in meta-analysis, embracing the idea that studies are likely to vary with one another even when they are all reportedly testing the same effect size. Random effects meta-analysis breaks down the variance between included studies into two parts: (1) within-study variance and (2) between-study variance. Within-study variance is based on differences in sample size between studies: Like a fixed-effect meta-analysis, random effects meta-analysis also weights studies with larger sample sizes relatively more than studies with smaller sample sizes. Unlike a fixed-effect meta, random effects meta does NOT assume that all studies are providing a test of the same 'true' (Fixed) effect. This is where the between-studies variance comes in and is the main reason why studies are weighted differently in fixed effect versus random effects meta-analysis.

A random effects meta-analysis works differently to a fixed-effect meta-analysis because it assumes that the 'true' effect size may vary between studies following a normal distribution and any meta-analysis pools only a *random* selection of tests of the range of true effects. Included studies only represent a random selection of all the tests that *could* have been performed. Such an approach acknowledges that the effect size in any individual study may vary because of factors like where the study was conducted, how data was collected (online or in person), how constructs or outcomes are measured, and so on. So in a random effects model, weighting is based on both the sampling error for each study (the within-study variance) as well as there being true variation between each study effect size and the overall effect, because the overall effect is the average of a *range* of true effects (the between-studies variance).

Meta-analysis works out the distance from the overall effect size to each individual effect size. To do this we need to calculate the variance of the distribution of true effects across studies (Tau^2) and the standard deviation of the distribution of true effects across studies (Tau). If you go to the outputs you generated in Chap. 9 you'll see that MAJOR outputs Tau and Tau^2 values for these meta-analyses.

In a random effects meta-analysis, you combine within-study variance, calculated as the inverse of the variance for each study (see Table 11.1) with between-studies variance, which is based on Tau^2. The formula for Tau^2 is not as intuitive as working out the inverse of the variance, which makes explaining the between-studies variance more challenging. If you are interested, I recommend working through Borenstein et al.'s (2021) examples, which are clear but require you to work through formulae. Regardless of whether you want to know how to calculate Tau^2 or not, the important thing is that including Tau^2 in the weighting of studies, alongside the within-studies variance, can make a difference between the weightings assigned to each included study and effect the overall effect size as we will see in the next section.

How Do Results Differ Between Fixed-Effect and Random Effects Meta-Analysis?

To illustrate how results change depending on whether you run a fixed-effect or random effects meta-analysis, I'm going to revisit the analysis I did in Chap. 9; it's advisable to have the output for Chap. 9 available when working through this comparison, so, if you haven't generated that output yet, go back and run the meta-analysis in Chap. 9 before reading on. I've included the output for the correlational meta-analysis, using the default model for MAJOR (Restricted Maximum-Likelihood Model) a random-effects model, in Fig. 11.2 and what happens when you change the model estimation to Fixed-Effect in Fig. 11.3. I've summarised results from the two methods in Table 11.2 to allow for a side-by-side comparison.

Let's talk through similarities and differences.

Similarities in Results Between Random Effects and Fixed-Effect Meta-Analyses

The effect size (correlation) is large-sized in both analyses, $r_+ = 0.55$ vs $r_+ = 0.51$, respectively, with both Z values being significant, indicating this effect size is significantly different from zero. Both I^2 values show high heterogeneity between

Correlation Coefficients

Random-Effects Model (k = 10)

	Estimate	se	Z	p	CI Lower Bound	CI Upper Bound
Intercept	0.546	0.0662	8.24	<.001	0.416	0.676
	.	.	.	.	.	.

Note. Tau^2 Estimator: Restricted Maximum-Likelihood

[3]

Heterogeneity Statistics

Tau	Tau^2	I^2	H^2	R^2	df	Q	p
0.192	0.0368 (SE= 0.0206)	91.04%	11.156	.	9.000	76.883	<.001

Fig. 11.2 Random-effects (Restricted Maximum-Likelihood) model output

Correlation Coefficients

Fixed-Effects Model (k = 10)

	Estimate	se	Z	p	CI Lower Bound	CI Upper Bound
Intercept	0.505	0.0165	30.7	<.001	0.473	0.537
	.	.	.	.	.	.

[3]

Heterogeneity Statistics

Tau	Tau^2	I^2	H^2	R^2	df	Q	p
0.000	0 (SE= NA)	88.29%	8.543	.	9.000	76.883	<.001

Fig. 11.3 Fixed-effect model output

studies' correlations. Importantly, the Q values, and their associated p values, are identical, which tells you that in random-effects meta-analysis, the Q test is based on a fixed-effect analysis (see Chap. 12).

Differences in Results Between Fixed-Effect and Random Effects Meta-Analyses

Although the effect sizes are both large-sized, they are not identical, which is due to how studies are weighted in each type of meta-analysis. Hinting at this difference you can see that the confidence intervals are narrower for the fixed-effect [0.47;

Table 11.2 Comparison of random effects and fixed-effect outputs

Statistics	Random-effects model	Fixed-effect model
Effect size (estimate)	0.546	0.505
Standard error	0.0662	0.0165
Z	8.24	30.7
p	< 0.001	< 0.001
Lower CI	0.416	0.473
Upper CI	0.676	0.537
Tau	0.192	0
Tau^2	0.0368	0
I^2	91.04	88.29
df	9	9
Q	76.883	76.883
p	< 0.001	< 0.001

0.54] vs the random effects [0.42; 0.68] model, and the Z value is almost 4 times bigger in the fixed effect meta. Tau values are only reported for the random effects analysis because they are not required in a fixed-effect meta-analysis (see above).

As stated above, a fixed-effect model assumes that the studies are testing the same effect size. So, the ten studies we meta-analysed mainly differ in how many people were recruited. A consequence of making this assumption is that you do not, in statistical terms, need to account for other sources of variance between studies, which means your analysis is, for want of a better term, more confident ☺. Less consideration of variation between studies leads you to believe that the range of possible values (confidence intervals) for the correlation is narrower. I'll end by noting that in interpretation terms, there's little difference between the models. Both estimates are for a large-sized correlation between intentions and behaviour, both are significant, the confidence intervals are quite similar, and both estimates show heterogeneity.

What does differentiate a fixed-effect from a random effects model is how each model *weights* the included studies. I'll use Forest plots to explain this point.

Before reading any further, please go back to the Model estimation tab and change your analysis back to Restricted Maximum Likelihood

How Do Fixed-Effect and Random-Effects Meta-Analyses Weight Studies?

In the Plots tab, click on the Model Fitting Weights, and your forest plot for a Restricted Maximum Likelihood model should look like Fig. 11.4:

This forest plot displays how much each study is weighted in the overall effect size. The weight of each study is reported in percentage terms that sum to 100; because the ten studies are used to generate the overall weight, the sum of their

Forest Plot

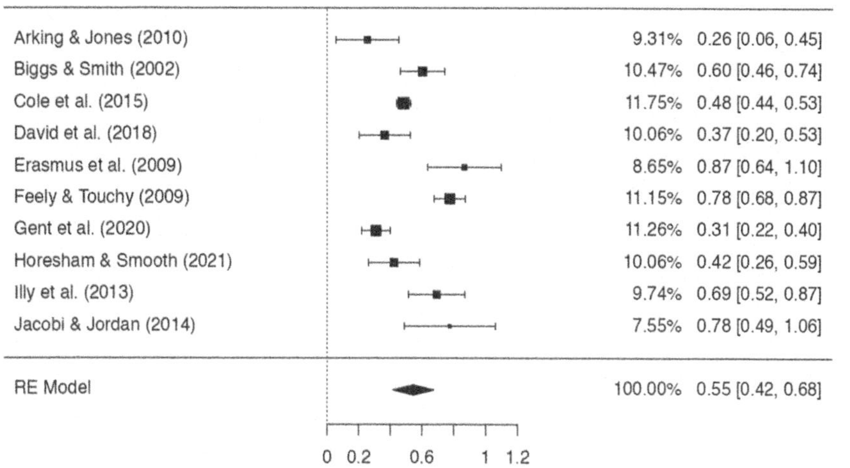

Fig. 11.4 Forest plot showing study weightings applying a random-effects (Restricted Maximum-Likelihood) model

weightings must add up to 100%. Cole et al. (2015), which has the largest sample size, also has the largest weighting (11.75%), while Jacobi and Jordan (2014), which has the smallest sample size, has the smallest weighting (7.55%). Weightings are quite similar sized, ranging from 7.55% to 11.75%. Now, change your model estimator to Fixed-Effect. You will end up with Fig. 11.5:

Look at the weightings again: Cole et al. (2015) now has a weighting of 54.05%, while Jacobi and Jordan (2014) is only 1.27%! In a fixed-effect meta-analysis, sample size drives weighting. This helps to explain why the overall correlation is lower for the fixed-effect meta than the random effects meta—Cole et al.'s (2015) sample size means its correlation exerts greater weight (influence) on the overall correlation in the fixed-effect vs the random effects model.

Hopefully you can see from the weightings in the two screenshots why results for the overall effect size differ depending on whether you use a random-effects or fixed-effect method. The remainder of the output is broadly similar for both models; the publication bias statistics are identical for random effects and fixed effect meta-analyses because they are based on standard errors that are relative to the overall effect size (see Chap. 13). The funnel plots do look slightly different, which I believe reflects the wider funnel in the random effects model.

Forest Plot

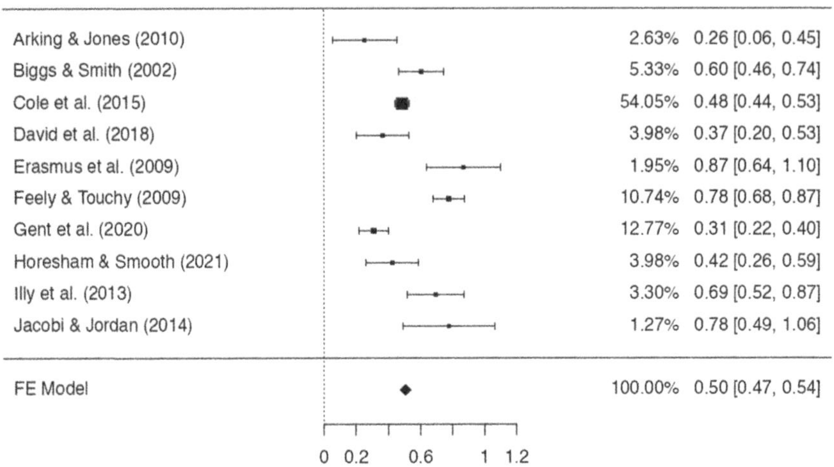

Fig. 11.5 Forest plot showing study weightings applying a fixed-effect model

Why I Prefer Random Effects Meta-Analysis

Random effects meta-analysis is a methodology that embraces the idea studies are likely to vary with one another in both known (measured) and unknown (unmeasured) ways, even when they are all, in theory, testing the same effect size. When studies are conducted, there is often a lack of consensus between research teams on aspects of study design, measurement, analytic approach, et cetera. So, even in Cooke et al. (2016), where studies were purportedly all testing the same theory relationships, and should have used similar designs and measures, we coded a range of factors that differed between studies.

Some of the differences between studies reflect choices made by research teams, such as, the age of the sample recruited. Most researchers tested theory relationships in young adults, a handful in adolescents. When you have a known (measured) factor that differs between studies, and enough cases of each level of the factor, you can conduct a moderator analysis (see Chap. 12) to compare effect sizes at different levels of this factor, that is, compare attitude–intention relationships for adolescents and adults as we did. Often, you'll be aware of these differences before you conduct the systematic review which informs the meta-analysis, and therefore it's best practice to add this information to your pre-registered protocol on either PROSPERO or the Open Science Framework. Sometimes, however, moderators come about only once you have completed data extraction.

For instance, we found across our 44 samples that researchers had reported 20 different definitions of alcohol consumption patterns!!! This lack of consensus in drinking definitions reflects a genuine lack of consensus in the alcohol literature, in my opinion. We adopted a liberal approach and included all the studies, which is OK when you adopt a random effects model but seems problematic to me if you were to run a fixed-effect meta-analysis because the research teams were not setting out to run broadly similar studies that differed only in sample size. We imposed some order on results by coding the different definitions and then running moderator analyses based on these codes (see Chap. 15 for more).

So far, we've only considered differences between included studies in things we know about (i.e. that have been measured and reported in the papers). What about differences between studies in things we **don't know** about, reminding us of Donald Rumsfeld's infamous 'Unknown, Unknowns' quote? There are likely to be a range of differences between studies that are unknown and potentially unknowable to the meta-analyst. Some of these reflect random variation in methods, others relate to more prosaic issues such as how well participants understood the questions they were answering and how valid the measures were.

The main reason I prefer to run random effects meta-analysis over fixed-effect meta-analysis is that I don't believe that psychological studies are run consistently across research teams. Most of the time when I conduct a meta-analysis, I'm dealing with papers that can seem to have limited awareness of the wider research literature, especially concerning a lack of consensus on measures of variables and outcomes and definitions of phenomena. While I do not think researchers are deliberately failing to standardise their methods, I'm all too familiar with papers in my research area doing things like creating their own measures of a construct, despite validated scales being available (see Cooke, 2021 for a discussion of this issue), and I have no idea if recruitment methods for psychology survey studies affect relationships nor how well samples that underrepresent groups generalise. In short, because it is rare for you as a meta-analyst to pool results from studies that have been conducted under highly controlled situations, I believe it makes it tough to justify using a fixed-effect analysis and believing that all that matters is sample size. Random effects methods reflect my experience of psychological research and that's why I use them.

Summary

Having compared fixed-effect and random effects meta-analysis in this chapter, in the next chapter, I'll go on to discuss how you can use moderator (sub-group) analyses to investigate heterogeneity between included studies.

References

Borenstein, M., Hedges, L. V., Higgins, J., & Rothstein, H. R. (2021). *Introduction to meta-analysis* (2nd ed.). Wiley.

Cooke, R. (2021). Psychological theories of alcohol consumption. In R. Cooke, D. Conroy, E. L. Davies, M. S. Hagger, & R. O. de Visser (Eds.), *The Palgrave handbook of psychological perspectives on alcohol consumption* (pp. 25–50). Springer International Publishing. https://doi.org/10.1007/978-3-030-66941-6_2

Cooke, R., Dahdah, M., Norman, P., & French, D. P. (2016). How well does the theory of planned behaviour predict alcohol consumption? A systematic review and meta-analysis. *Health Psychology Review, 10*, 148–167. https://doi.org/10.1080/17437199.2014.947547

Cooke, R., & French, D. P. (2008). How well do the theory of reasoned action and theory of planned behaviour predict intentions and attendance at screening programmes? A meta-analysis. *Psychology & Health, 23*(7), 745–765. https://doi.org/10.1080/08870440701544437

Cooke, R., McEwan, H., & Norman, P. (2023). The effect of forming implementation intentions on alcohol consumption: A systematic review and meta-analysis. *Drug and Alcohol Review, 42*, 68–80. https://doi.org/10.1111/dar.13553

Cooke, R., & Sheeran, P. (2004). Moderation of cognition-intention and cognition-behaviour relations: A meta-analysis of properties of variables from the theory of planned behaviour. *The British Journal of Social Psychology, 43*(Pt 2), 159–186. https://doi.org/10.1348/0144666041501688

Moderator (Sub-group) Analyses

12

Heterogeneity Between Effect Sizes—a Challenge to Precision in Meta-Analysis

A key aim of meta-analysis is to provide a precise estimate of an effect size by pooling results across studies. However, it is common for there to be substantial heterogeneity between effect sizes reported in the psychological literature. Indeed, the only examples from my meta-analyses where we found a lack of heterogeneity in an overall effect size was for the null effect size difference of implementation intentions on heavy episodic drinking reported in Cooke et al. (2023) and the null correlation between perceived control and drinking behaviour in Cooke et al. (2016). All other overall meta-analyses I've computed and published have shown significant heterogeneity, so, you should be prepared for this when conducting your meta-analysis as heterogeneity is likely.

The aim of this chapter is to take you through the process of thinking about moderators from the inception of your meta-analysis through to interpretation of moderator analyses. I'll begin by defining moderators before moving on to getting you to think about moderators when creating your protocol for your review. Next, I'll use examples from my meta-analyses to show how moderators can reduce heterogeneity between studies by creating sub-sets of studies that, by possessing similar sample or methodological characteristics, report similar effect sizes. Finally, I'll discuss how I've run moderator analyses in software packages previously to advise you about how to do this yourself.

Statistics Used to Test Heterogeneity in Meta-Analysis

Three statistics are output following meta-analyses as indicators of heterogeneity: Q (chi-square) test, Tau^2, and I^2. Each statistic provides different information. The Q test measures the weighted standard deviations for included studies; Tau^2 is the

R. Cooke, *Meta-Analysis for Psychologists*,
https://doi.org/10.1007/978-3-031-73773-2_12

between studies variance, (see Chap. 11); I^2 represents the ratio of true heterogeneity to total observed variation.

In a random-effects meta-analysis, we assume that the 'true' effect size can vary between studies and weight studies according to this principle (see Chap. 11). This means there is naturally going to be variability in effect sizes because unlike with a fixed-effect meta, you accept the possibility that the true effect size can vary. So, part of heterogeneity in overall effect sizes is a consequence of this between-study variance in true effect sizes. There is also heterogeneity due to sampling (within-study) error, which reflects differences between studies in sample sizes. When thinking about heterogeneity in overall effect sizes, we seek to partition it into between-studies and within-studies components. I'll start by discussing the Q statistic which helps understand the within-studies component.

The Q statistic represents the ratio of observed variation to within-study error. To compute Q, you calculate the deviation of each effect size from the overall effect size, square it, weight it by the inverse variance (see Table 11.1) and then sum the results. This produces a weighted sum of squares or Q value. Because you are subtracting each effect size from the overall effect size you are creating a standardised measure, which means it does not matter what scale your effect size is on. Once we have computed our Q value, we next work out our expected value under the assumption that all studies share a common effect size. This is simply the degrees of freedom, that is, the number of studies (K) – 1. So, if you have ten studies, your degrees of freedom would be nine.

We now have an observed weighted sum of squares (i.e. the Q value) and an expected weighted sum of squares (degrees of freedom). If we subtract the degrees of freedom from the Q value, we get the excess variation to answer the question "Does observed variation between studies effect sizes, exceed what we would expect?" If your Q value exceeds your degrees of freedom, this tells you that you have more variation between studies than would be expected. This means that Q is dependent on the number of studies you include in your meta-analysis. So, a non-significant Q value indicates a lack of heterogeneity between effect sizes because the variation of the effect sizes is less than we would expect based on how many effect sizes are included in the meta; more effect sizes = more expected variation.

When you see a Q value in a meta-analytic output, it is accompanied by a p value, which follows the tradition common to psychology of being significant at $p < 0.05$ (or lower) and non-significant if $p > 0.05$. For example, the Q value is significant for the meta-analysis of correlations in Chap. 9, but not for the meta-analysis of effect size differences in Chap. 10. The Q test is testing the null hypothesis that all studies share a common effect size, reasoning that is more in keeping with a fixed-effect than random-effects meta-analysis (and hence why the Q values are the same in Table 11.2). So, a significant Q suggests studies vary in their 'true' effect size. However, as Borenstein et al. (2021) note, a non-significant Q value does not imply that effect sizes are similar (or homogenous). The lack of significance may be due to low power, which is likely with a small number of studies and/or small sample sizes.

While Q focuses on within-study variation, following the assumption that all included studies have the same 'true' effect size, Tau^2 is a metric of variance in the 'true' effect sizes. This value is calculated by subtracting the Q value (weighted sum of squares) from the degrees of freedom ($K - 1$) then dividing the result by the sum of the study weights minus the sum of the study weights squared divided by the sum of the study weights. All this means our standardised measure of dispersion, Q, has been turned back into the scale used in the meta-analysis and making it an average of squared deviations. Tau^2 reflects the absolute amount of variance in the scale.

Because Tau^2 is based partially on Q, this means it can be zero if Q is less than the degrees of freedom. In most meta-analyses, this is not the case, however, so Tau^2 is computed. There are two factors that influence Tau^2 values (a) excess variation and (b) the metric used to generate the effect size. As excess variation (Q—degrees of freedom) increases, so does Tau^2. The other cause of higher Tau^2 values is where the absolute amount of variance in the set of studies is higher. So, meta-analyses that include studies with wider confidence intervals, indicating smaller sample sizes, will have a higher absolute amount of variance, relative to meta-analyses with studies containing narrower confidence intervals.

In my previous meta-analyses, I've never reported Tau^2 as I don't think it is a particularly intuitive statistic to report to when understanding heterogeneity. Instead, I recommend generating prediction intervals (see Chap. 14) on forest plots, which are based on Tau^2 to provide a more intuitive measure of heterogeneity in 'true' effect sizes.

The final measure of heterogeneity is the I^2 statistic. Higgins (2003) proposed this as measure of inconsistency in effect sizes. The I^2 value represents the proportion of observed variance that reflects real differences in effect sizes. You calculate I^2 based on the subtracting Q from the degrees of freedom, dividing this value by Q and then multiplying by 100, to give you a percentage value (I^2 is bounded from 0% to 100%). The formula gives you the ratio of excess dispersion (Q—degrees of freedom) to total dispersion (Q). Put another way, it is the ratio of variance between studies relative to total variance.

As I^2 is based on Q values, it is perhaps not surprising that as Q increases so does I^2. It reflects the extent of overlap of confidence intervals and can be seen as a measure of inconsistency across study findings; it does not tell you anything about the 'true' effects for studies, however. One difference between I^2 and Q is that I^2 is not affected by the number of studies in the way Q is. Borenstein et al. (2021) argue that I^2 can be used to determine what proportion of observed variance is real. Low I^2 values suggest observed variance is mostly spurious, whereas moderate and higher values of I^2 imply that there are factors that underlie differences between studies' effect sizes. This is where moderator (sub-group) analyses come in.

Introduction to Moderator (Sub-group) Analyses

When I first started thinking about meta-analysis, I was encouraged to think about variables that might moderate the correlations included in my meta-analysis. Indeed, Cooke and Sheeran (2004) literally used meta-analysis to test moderators of theory of planned behaviour relationships (e.g. attitude–intention; intention–behaviour) using properties of cognition (e.g. how accessible attitudes and intentions are in memory; how stable intentions are over time). Hence, considering moderators when planning a meta-analysis is so engrained in my thinking that I struggle to conceive of conducting a meta-analysis without specifying moderators a priori.

I'll use Sheeran and Orbell's (1998) meta-analysis as an example of how to identify factors that might moderate an overall effect size in meta-analysis. Six factors—sexual orientation; gender; sample age; time interval; intention versus expectation; steady versus casual partners—were proposed as potential moderators of the size of the relationship between condom use intentions and condom use. We can split these into sample and methodological moderators.

Sample moderators are factors that capture differences between studies in samples recruited. Sexual orientation, gender, sample age, and casual versus steady partners are all sample moderators as they reflect characteristics of the samples recruited. Methodological moderators capture methodological differences between included studies: Time interval (i.e. the gap between measurement of intentions and measurement of condom use) and intention versus expectation are both methodological moderators.

Sampling factors are sometimes outside the control of researchers conducting primary studies; you might aim to recruit a sample with roughly equal numbers of younger and older participants but end up with more of one group than the other. In contrast, methodological factors tend to reflect decisions made by the researchers conducting primary studies. The two methodological moderators mentioned above highlight this principle in action; researchers decided how big the time interval between measures of intentions and condom use was and if they wanted to measure intentions or expectations.

Sheeran and Orbell (1998) reported mixed evidence for the effect of the six moderators on their overall effect size of $r_+ = 0.44$ between intentions and condom use. Some moderators did not affect the overall effect size: the sample-weighted average correlation was $r_+ = 0.45$ for men and $r_+ = 0.44$ for women, while the sample-weighted average correlations for intention ($r_+ = 0.44$) and expectation ($r_+ = 0.43$) did not differ from one another either. The lack of difference due to moderators tells us that these variables do not offer effective explanations for heterogeneity in the overall effect size. A *lack* of difference in effect sizes between levels of a categorical moderator suggests that variation on this factor is not causing heterogeneity in the overall effect size. Other factors moderated the overall effect size: Adolescents reported weaker correlations ($r_+ = 0.25$) than older samples ($r_+ = 0.50$); the effect size was stronger over shorter time intervals (less than 10 weeks, $r_+ = 0.59$; more than 10 weeks $r_+ = 0.33$). The former result suggests that younger samples intentions are less likely to be enacted than older samples, while the latter result implies that intentions change over time, something I found in my PhD. Finally, the moderating effect of sexual orientation could not be tested due to a lack of studies, an issue we'll return to later in the chapter.

How to Identify Moderators When Writing the Protocol for Your Meta-Analysis

I think it's relatively easy to come up with sample factors a priori—in most meta-analyses you can assume that gender (or some aspect of sex or classification system) might influence results, and I've already discussed age as another sample moderator. Conversely, sexual orientation and/or casual versus steady partner are not moderators that would be suitable in meta-analyses of other topics. Identifying methodological factors a priori takes a bit more thought but can still be done—time interval between measurement is something that could easily affect the size of a correlation or the effect size difference, so, might be a viable candidate for any meta-analysis.

Other methodological factors are likely to be specific to your meta-analysis. Unlike in the late 1990s, we don't spend much time thinking about behavioural intentions vs behavioural expectations anymore, but there will be methodological factors that are relevant to your meta-analysis that are worth considering. For example, we knew there were different types of implementation intention interventions—if-then plans, self-affirmation implementation intentions, volitional help sheets—when we pre-registered Cooke et al. (2023). During data extraction, we also found that there were mental contrasting implementation intentions.

Specifying moderators in advance is a balance between knowing what factors are likely to affect results and reflecting on the suitability of moderators that are tested in many meta-analyses. There is no penalty for proposing moderator analyses a priori that prove impossible to conduct. Indeed, when we had finished coding studies for Cooke et al. (2023), we only had sufficient studies to compare effect size differences for studies that used if-then plans or volitional help sheet. Box 12.1 contains some tips about methodological moderators.

Box 12.1 Thinking About Methodological Moderators When thinking about your meta-analysis, there's no harm in reading through published meta-analyses in your area, or related areas, to identify potential moderators. Some will make sense for your meta and some will not. One thing I would recommend, however, is you reflect on the methodology used to conduct studies you are likely to include in your meta-analysis. If you are looking at experimental designs or interventions, then think about design issues like follow-up periods, content of material received by intervention and control groups, think about how the outcomes you are interested in are likely to be measured—is there a commonly used scale to assess educational achievement, or pain, or a measure of personality everyone uses? Maybe there's a whole range of different measures. Alternatively, if you plan to run a meta-analysis of correlations, think about how constructs are measured (using a validated scale), are constructs representing a theory or model, and the gap between measurement points (if there is one). Whatever the case, thinking about the methods used in your literature is a good use of your time prior to beginning your meta-analysis as it will help you write your protocol and can prepare you for what's to come.

How Moderator Analysis Works in Meta-Analysis

In essence, moderator analysis is testing to see if an effect size—be it a correlation or an effect size difference in an outcome—is moderated by another factor. In primary papers, moderation takes the form of seeing if dichotomous variables like gender (female or male), categorical variables like age (young, middle-aged, older aged), or continuous variables like past behaviour affect the magnitude of correlations between variables or the effect size difference in an outcome.

For example, in Cooke and Sheeran (2013), we found that the more stable one's intentions are over time, the stronger the relationship between intentions and behaviour. We used a method called Simple Slopes analysis (Aiken & West, 1991) to plot the relationship between the two variables at three levels of the moderator: low stability; medium stability; high stability. When you run moderation, rather than having one effect size for everyone, you are creating sub-groups and calculating the effect size at different levels of the moderator (low, medium, high; young, old) to see if the effect size differs between levels.

A key difference when thinking about moderation in meta-analysis is that because you are conducting a secondary analysis, you don't have access to the raw data used to generate the summary statistics used in the paper. This means moderation typically relies on simpler tests, like Z or Q tests, to compare sub-groups of studies. In my experience, meta-analyses tend to involve dichotomous (binary) or categorical moderator analyses more than continuous moderator analyses. I'll discuss these different types in the next section.

Dichotomous (Binary) Moderator Variables

With dichotomous (binary) moderator analyses, you run separate meta-analyses for studies depending on which level of the moderator they represent, that is, all studies that reported correlations between expectations–condom use are meta-analysed, with the intention–condom use correlations separated out and meta-analysed together. Once you have done this, you can run Fisher's (1921) Z test to see if the correlations significantly differed from one another. The Z test checks the idea that two correlations are drawn from independent samples, in other words, that they significantly differ from one another.

In Cooke and Sheeran (2004), I computed overall effect sizes for high versus low levels of properties of cognitions (temporal stability, accessibility, etc.) then ran Z tests to see if they differed from one another. Alternatively, in Cooke et al. (2023), we tested the idea that sample type (community, university) moderated the effect size difference in weekly alcohol consumption. We found a larger effect size difference in consumption for community samples ($d_+ = -0.38$) compared with university samples ($d_+ = -0.04$). We used the Q test, which is more typically used with categorical moderator variables, to confirm that these effect size differences significantly differed from one another. As an aside, both community and university effect size differences were not heterogeneous, suggesting that coding studies based on the sample recruited created sub-sets of studies that found similar effect sizes.

Categorical Moderator Variables

Any variable with more than two levels is classed as a categorical moderator, which are analysed using the Q test. This statistic seeks to test the idea that there is significant (overall) heterogeneity between all sub-groups of studies in your meta-analysis. If there is overall heterogeneity in the overall test, this means that your effect sizes for your categories differ from one another.

In Cooke and French (2008), we found evidence of heterogeneity in each of the five effect sizes representing theory of planned behaviour relationships we meta-analysed. Type of screening test was a categorical moderator we tested to try and reduce heterogeneity between studies. This moderator had six levels: cervical smear, colorectal cancer, genetic test, health check, mammography, and prenatal. Type of screening test moderated four of the overall effect sizes, suggesting that type of screening is an important factor to consider when testing theory relationships. When categorical moderators are significant, you can use pairwise Z tests to identify pairs of sub-groups where these differences exist. The fifth relationship, between perceived behavioural control and behaviour, however, showed no effect of this moderator indicating that the correlation between control and behaviour was similar regardless of screening type. Moderators do not always moderate effect sizes!

In each of the significant analyses, you see a difference between the heterogeneity statistic (Q) for the overall effect size (i.e. the attitude–intention relationship across all screening studies) and the moderator results (i.e. the attitude–intention relationship computed separately for cervical smear studies, colorectal cancer, genetic test, health check, mammography, and prenatal studies). For example, overall, heterogeneity for the attitude–intention relationship was chi-square = 737.96; after coding studies into type of screening test, chi-square reduced to 345.32. This suggests that grouping effect sizes by type of screening test has accounted for some of the heterogeneity between effect sizes. However, you are not formally testing anything using this method, so be wary about the claims you make. Formal tests of effects of moderators exist and are discussed in the 'Testing Multiple Moderators Simultaneously' section.

The other thing to note regards the non-significant moderation for the perceived behavioural control–behaviour relationship. Heterogeneity between studies in the overall meta for this effect size was significant but also the lowest of the five relationships (chi-square = 58.13); in the moderated analysis, the value was non-significant chi-square = 6.86. Two things to comment on. First, because the overall heterogeneity was lower for this relationship, relative to the other relationships, there was less heterogeneity to explain in absolute terms. Second, even though there was less heterogeneity, type of screening test did not appear to account for this heterogeneity, and as a result, this moderator did not help explain the overall heterogeneity for this relationship. When this happens, it's reasonable to look at alternative moderators to explain overall heterogeneity.

Continuous Moderator Variables

When you have a continuous moderator variable, like time interval between measurements, you can either transform it into categorical variable like Sheeran and Orbell (1998) did by coding studies based on a median split for the intervals, or use a technique called meta-regression to plot the effects of the moderator on the effect size. In Cooke et al. (2023), we found evidence that time interval was a significant moderator of effect sizes, such that studies with shorter intervals between measures showed larger effect size differences, although this effect was small. In Comprehensive Meta-Analysis, you can generate meta-regression plots to visualise these effects.

Testing Multiple Moderators Simultaneously

In Sheeran and Orbell (1998), age and time interval were both significant moderators of the overall effect size, which begs the question of whether the factors might interact with one another. They dealt with this issue by creating sub-sub-groups by crossing the levels of each factor with one another: that is, adolescent short-term and long-term intervals; older short-term and long-term intervals. While an eminently practical solution, this approach relies on their being sufficient papers in each cell of this design to test differences and does not provide a formal test of each moderator against the other moderator because you have split the factors into four groups, reducing the power of your analysis.

An alternative approach with more statistical power is to run a mixed effects meta-analysis, which is like a multiple regression in a primary paper. After coding moderators as variables in your dataset (see below), you ask your software package to test the effects of each moderator simultaneously. For example, in Cooke et al. (2023), we had three significant moderators: time frame (continuous); sample type (dichotomous); mode of delivery (dichotomous). The mixed-effect meta-analysis found that sample type and time interval were both significant moderators and that the heterogeneity in the (overall) effect size reduced to non-significance in the presence of these moderators. In other words, when we accounted for the effects of time interval, sample type, and mode of delivery, the overall effect size was now homogenous. This suggests that these moderators provide important clues as to why effect sizes differed in the overall analysis. This analysis generates questions for future research questions too.

What About When Moderators Are Confounded with One Another?

One of the reasons I think that mode of delivery was not a significant moderator in the mixed effect meta-analysis is that it was likely confounded with sample type; almost all our university samples received their intervention via online mode of delivery, while all of our community samples received their intervention via paper mode of delivery. Hence, sample type and mode of delivery were confounded because we cannot disentangle the effect of sample from the mode of delivery. If we had been able to identify studies that delivered interventions to community samples online, along with more studies delivering interventions via paper to university samples, we might have been able to disentangle the effects of the two moderators, but we would have been in a similar position to Paschal and Sheena in needing enough studies for each cell of the comparison.

I think the simplest solution to confounded moderator variables is to conduct primary studies to test the factors experimentally. Remember that in meta-analysis we are using the endpoint of a set of research studies, their findings to pool results together. When we find heterogeneity in effect sizes, and that methodological or sample variables as putative moderators of this heterogeneity, it can mean a lack of research attention to an issue, such as a lack of studies delivering implementation intentions interventions to community samples online. While we could wait for more studies to address this issue in a future meta-analysis, it strikes me that a better idea would be to run those studies using the meta-analysis to guide our research plans. Having thoroughly discussed moderator analyses, I'll now discuss ways to run moderator analyses in software packages.

How to Perform Moderator Analyses as Part of a Meta-Analysis

The first step in any moderator analysis comes during data extraction. When extracting key information from study characteristics, for example, author names, country of study, demographics, you also code included studies for moderator variables.

I'll give two examples of how I did this for my meta-analyses:

- In Cooke et al. (2016), we coded studies as having either adolescent or adult samples: Studies were coded as 1 if an adolescent sample was recruited or 2 if an adult sample was recruited.

- In Cooke et al. (2023), we coded studies as testing either an if-then implementation intention, a self-affirmation implementation intention, or a volitional help sheet. Studies that used if-then plans were coded as 1, self-affirmation implementation intentions as 2, and volitional help sheets as 3.

The next stage is to create variables to add the information into your dataset. Create a new variable, give it a name that reflects what it represents and decide what type of variable it is going to be: dichotomous; categorical; continuous. Some programmes, including Comprehensive Meta-Analysis and metafor, are happy for you to enter either text, to represent the categories, or numbers that represent groups. Continuous moderators must be entered as numerical information. Jamovi prefers numerical values.

Before I go any further, I must admit that although MAJOR is a great package for introducing meta-analysis, it is limited when it comes to running moderator analyses. It does not offer as much flexibility in moderator analyses as either Comprehensive Meta Analysis (which I used in Cooke et al., 2016) or metafor (which I used in Cooke et al., 2023). Currently, MAJOR allows you to test the effect of a single moderator on your overall effect size and this variable can be either categorical (including dichotomous variables) or continuous. However, there does not seem to be any way to run separate meta-analyses by level of categorical moderator, as it is possible to do in Comprehensive Meta Analysis and metafor, other than creating separate datasets based on the levels of the moderator, that is, a dataset containing data for only the community samples or only the university samples. As a result, it's hard to recommend using MAJOR to test moderation in your meta-analysis currently. I will run a basic analysis to show you what is possible.

Running a Moderator Analysis in Jamovi

We're going to use the dataset from Chap. 9 as our example because results for this meta-analysis indicated significant heterogeneity. In brief, we found an overall correlation that was large-sized ($r_+ = 0.55$), with evidence of high heterogeneity $I^2 = 91.04$, $Q = 76.88$, $p < 0.001$. We can test the impact of a moderator on the I^2 and Q values by entering it into the moderator box in the meta-analysis in MAJOR. Reductions in these values imply that by coding studies using a moderator, we have accounted for some of the heterogeneity between studies in the effect size. I've added the moderator "Time Interval" to the dataset, (see Table 12.1). Copy this information into your dataset and then add the variable to the Moderator box in your meta-analysis. Your output will look like Fig. 12.1:

The output shows the effect of time interval as a moderator of correlations between measures of drinking intentions and drinking behaviour (1 = 6-month gap between measures; 2 = 3–5-month gap; 3 = less than a 3-month gap) in the top table, which is a significant result. The bottom table shows the heterogeneity statistics covered at the beginning of the chapter: Q, I^2, and Tau^2. Relative to the meta-analysis

Table 12.1 Correlations between drinking intentions and behaviour with sample sizes and time interval as a moderator

Study authors + year	Correlation (r)	Sample size (N)	Time interval
Arking and Jones (2010)	0.25	100	1
Biggs and Smith (2002)	0.54	200	2
Cole et al. (2015)	0.45	2000	2
David et al. (2018)	0.35	150	1
Erasmus et al. (2009)	0.70	75	2
Feely and Touchy (2007)	0.65	400	3
Gent et al. (2020)	0.30	475	1
Horseham and Smooth (2021)	0.40	150	2
Illy et al. (2013)	0.60	125	3
Jacobi and Jordan (2014)	0.65	50	3

Correlation Coefficients

Mixed-Effects Model (k = 10)

	Estimate	se	Z	p	CI Lower Bound	CI Upper Bound
Intercept	0.0956	0.0765	1.25	0.211	−0.054	0.246
Moderator	0.2193	0.0367	5.97	<.001	0.147	0.291

Note. Tau² Estimator: Restricted Maximum-Likelihood

[3]

Heterogeneity Statistics

Tau	Tau²	I²	H²	R²	df	Q	p
0.049	0.0024 (SE= 0.0034)	39.45%	1.652	93.4%	9.000	15.471	0.051

Fig. 12.1 Output from moderator analysis in MAJOR

without the moderator, Q and I^2 values have reduced, which suggests that some of the heterogeneity between studies has been accounted for. The Q value is no longer significant, but recall that we can only infer a meaningful result from a significant Q value, not from a non-significant value, so caution is urged here.

Some Cautionary Notes About Moderator Analyses

I want to end this chapter with a section covering a few issues for you to consider when running moderator analyses. A key issue is determining how many papers you need to run a moderator analysis. As Hagger (2022) succinctly puts it, the answer to the question of the minimum number of papers needed for any meta-analysis is simple, it's two! As Martin goes on to say, however, unless these two studies have used robust study designs, validated measures, et cetera, you can debate the value in pooling their results together. Even having more studies is not enough for some journal editors and reviewers; Cooke and French (2008), which contains meta-analyses based on $K = 33$ tests of attitude–intention and $K = 19$ tests of the intention–behaviour relationship, was labelled as 'premature' by a reviewer from the first journal we submitted it to, while we had to delay re-submission of Cooke et al. (2023) after rejection by the first journal having been told we needed more studies.

As there is no agreed-upon number of studies that is sufficient for a meta-analysis (see Chap. 2), you need to be cautious when running moderator analyses. In moderator analyses, you are splitting your sample of studies into sub-groups, which often produces even smaller sets of studies to meta-analyse. While there's no hard and fast rules about the numbers of studies needed for each level of your moderator variable, it's advisable to only run moderator analyses when you have more than two studies for each level and I feel more comfortable having more than this number of studies, usually four or five per level. In Cooke et al. (2023), we decided not to include self-affirmation implementation intention studies in our test of intervention type because we only had two of these studies, nor mental contrasting implementation intentions as we had only one study. We were wary about inferring too much from meta-analyses based on such numbers of studies. Ideally, you would have at least five studies for each level of your moderator, but the more the better, as we know that Q statistics are sensitive to the number of studies included.

Another issue to be aware of is that it is not always possible to code all included studies for every moderator. For example, in Cooke and French (2008), a paper on tuberculosis inoculation did not clearly fit within the categories for type of screening test moderator. Consequently, we left this paper out of the moderator analyses, which is a reason to be careful when comparing heterogeneity levels for overall analyses (with all studies included) with moderator analyses, where studies may be excluded. A further consequence of not being able to code all studies is that you will not always be able to include all moderators in your mixed-effects model. In Cooke et al. (2023), we only tested three of the four moderators in the mixed model because there were not enough self-affirmation implementation intention studies to include type of intervention in the analysis. This is akin to missing data for a variable in a primary analysis; if you have missing data for an individual on one variable, then that individual's data is excluded from the analysis. In meta-analysis, the same logic applies, but it is at the level of the study rather than the individual.

Summary

The aim of this chapter was to discuss running moderator analyses to address heterogeneity between effect sizes in meta-analysis. In the next chapter, we'll discuss how publication bias can affect meta-analytic results.

References

Aiken, L. S., & West, S. G. (1991). *Multiple regression: Testing and interpreting interactions*. SAGE.

Borenstein, M., Hedges, L. V., Higgins, J., & Rothstein, H. R. (2021). *Introduction to meta-analysis* (2nd ed.). Wiley.

Cooke, R., Dahdah, M., Norman, P., & French, D. P. (2016). How well does the theory of planned behaviour predict alcohol consumption? A systematic review and meta-analysis. *Health Psychology Review, 10*, 148–167. https://doi.org/10.1080/17437199.2014.947547

Cooke, R., & French, D. P. (2008). How well do the theory of reasoned action and theory of planned behaviour predict intentions and attendance at screening programmes? A meta-analysis. *Psychology & Health, 23*(7), 745–765. https://doi.org/10.1080/08870440701544437

Cooke, R., McEwan, H., & Norman, P. (2023). The effect of forming implementation intentions on alcohol consumption: A systematic review and meta-analysis. *Drug and Alcohol Review, 42*, 68–80. https://doi.org/10.1111/dar.13553

Cooke, R., & Sheeran, P. (2004). Moderation of cognition-intention and cognition-behaviour relations: A meta-analysis of properties of variables from the theory of planned behaviour. *The British Journal of Social Psychology, 43*(Pt 2), 159–186. https://doi.org/10.1348/0144666041501688

Cooke, R., & Sheeran, P. (2013). Properties of intention: Component structure and consequences for behavior, information processing, and resistance. *Journal of Applied Social Psychology, 43*(4), 749–760. https://doi.org/10.1111/jasp.12003

Fisher, R. A. (1921). On the probable error of a coefficient of correlation deduced from a small sample. *Metron, 1*, 3–32.

Hagger, M. S. (2022). Meta-analysis. *International Review of Sport and Exercise Psychology, 15*(1), 120–151. https://doi.org/10.1080/1750984X.2021.1966824

Higgins, J. P. T. (2003). Measuring inconsistency in meta-analyses. *BMJ, 327*(7414), 557–560. https://doi.org/10.1136/bmj.327.7414.557

Sheeran, P., & Orbell, S. (1998). Do intentions predict condom use? Meta-analysis and examination of six moderator variables. *British Journal of Social Psychology, 37*(2), 231–250. https://doi.org/10.1111/j.2044-8309.1998.tb01167.x

References

13 Publication Bias

What Is Publication Bias?

Publication bias is the tendency of journals to favour publication of papers that report significant findings (e.g. my intervention significantly reduced screen time) relative to papers that report non-significant findings (e.g. my intervention reduced screen time but not significantly) or null findings (e.g. my intervention had no effect on screen time). It's easy to see why publication bias happens; journal editors want to publish studies reporting exciting, novel significant findings in their journals because they know that such findings are more likely to garner the attention of the academic community and attract media interest than studies whose results appear more routine or humdrum. The irony is that the dictionary definition of good science is results that are routine or humdrum, that is, ones that replicate across contexts and target populations. Science should be replicable, with different teams of researchers able to find similar results when applying the same methods.

Unfortunately, publication bias has a pernicious effect on researchers; because they know that studies reporting significant findings are more likely to be published, they put more effort into getting studies that show significant findings published, often putting away non-significant findings in the metaphorical file drawer (Rosenthal, 1979). Alternatively, there is also the temptation to engage in dubious practices like p-hacking, where researchers play around with their datasets until they stumble upon a significant result, regardless of the meaningfulness of this result. Psychology as a discipline has a bad reputation for replicability of findings (Chambers, 2017). Psychologists typically don't like running the same study many times to confirm results replicate (because replications are also less likely to get published). Such bad practice is less common in other disciplines. Biochemists, for example, check their results with independent labs before publication. Physicists share results online. Psychologists are slowly starting to embrace Open Science practices, which will help address issues of replicability, so hopefully publication bias will become less of an issue over time. While it is beyond the scope of this book

R. Cooke, *Meta-Analysis for Psychologists*,
https://doi.org/10.1007/978-3-031-73773-2_13

to go into further detail about the concept of publication bias, we are covering this topic in the book because meta-analysis can play a role in identifying publication bias within research literatures.

Why Does Publication Bias Matter When Conducting a Meta-Analysis?

The main reason I run meta-analyses is to find a precise estimate of an effect size I'm interested in to allow me to answer research questions like "What is the direction and magnitude of the correlation between drinking intentions and drinking behaviour?" I want to know the answer to this question for various reasons, including to (1) know if the theoretical ideas I'm researching are supported across multiple studies; (2) be able to compare that effect size with effect sizes for other relationships; and (3) be able to estimate the sample size I need in future studies testing this effect size.

Because publication bias has the potential to undermine confidence in the results of meta-analyses, software packages for meta-analysis include statistical and graphical methods to help identify this bias. I covered these issues briefly in Chaps. 9 and 10 when discussing the output generated by MAJOR. In this chapter, I'll elaborate on what measures of publication bias mean in the next few pages.

Statistics Used to Identify Publication Bias in Meta-Analysis

Fail-Safe N Values

Rosenthal (1979) was one of the first researchers to draw attention to publication bias, coining the phrase 'the file-drawer problem' to cover the situation where non-significant results end up in a file-drawer. He also proposed a statistical test to estimate the extent of publication bias in a literature: Fail-Safe N values tell you the number of studies you would need to find, in addition to those you have included in your meta-analysis, that report null effect sizes (i.e. $r = 0.00$; $d = 0.00$) to undermine confidence in your results. I use examples to illustrate how Fail-Safe N works.

Let's imagine Terry locates 15 studies testing the correlation between physical activity attitudes and physical activity intentions. They meta-analyse the correlations generating a sample-weighted average correlation of $r_+ = 0.35$. Their Publication Bias Assessment table tells them they have a Fail-Safe N value of 100. This means that to undermine Terry's confidence in their results they would need to find 100 studies all with **null** correlations between attitudes and intention, *in addition* to the 15 studies they found, to undermine confidence that there is a significant correlation of the magnitude reported above. It's like asking 'How many studies that show no effect would I need to find to bring my overall effect size down to zero?' In this case, it would be 100 null studies. It is important to note that you interpret values relative to the number of studies you found to add context. If Terry finds 15 studies, it is unlikely he has missed 100 additional studies, and, that these all show null findings.

Alternatively, let's imagine Alex is interested in the difference between educational intervention and control groups on mathematical reasoning. They find 25 studies produce a pooled effect size difference of $d_+ = 0.55$, favouring the intervention group participants. Their Publication Bias Assessment table gives a Fail-Safe N value of 250. As in Terry's example, the same logic applies 'How many studies, all showing null effect size differences, would you need to find to bring my overall effect size down to zero?" In this case it is 250 studies. This gives Alex confidence in their findings; having systematically searched the literature and found 25 relevant studies, it's unlikely that they've failed to locate 250 null findings. This means they can be confident that their results are not unduly affected by missing results.

MAJOR allows you to choose between different Fail-Safe N Methods, including Rosenthal's (1979) and Orwin's (1983). Rosenthal's method is the default in MAJOR and he tells you how many null studies you would need to locate to reduce your effect size to zero. This method assumes you have a significant effect size, that could be reduced to non-significance, so, if you have a null result from your meta-analysis, I'm not sure there's much point in reporting Rosenthal's statistic because there's no effect to reduce. Borenstein et al. (2009) note several additional weaknesses with Rosenthal's method. First, it focuses on statistical significance, which tends to be of less interest in a meta-analysis where we are more focused on the direction and magnitude of the overall effect size (see Chap. 7). Second, the formula assumes that all missing studies report null effects. Missing studies could in principle report null, negative, positive effects, so this assumption is questionable at best; just because a study finds a positive effect does not guarantee it will be published and, alternatively, not all negative or null effects are absent from the published literature. Finally, the test is based on combining p values across studies, a common practice when Rosenthal published his work in 1979. It's more common nowadays to compute the overall effect size and then compute the p value.

Orwin's (1983) method tells you how many studies you need to reduce your effect size difference's magnitude from one category to another, that is, from a large effect size to a medium effect size. When evaluating interventions, such statistics can be used to guide as to how much confidence we should give our results. A large Orwin value serves to tell us that it would take a lot of null results to shift our view that we have, across studies, a medium effect size difference; not impossible, but not likely either. In contrast, a small Orwin value would suggest that our effect size is not as stable as we might like. An important consideration with Orwin's value is what magnitude of effect size are you starting with? In my experience, meta-analyses of correlations are more likely to be large or medium-sized than meta-analyses of effect size differences, which are more likely to be medium or small-sized. I think this reflects a simple idea; that it's easier to find evidence for a correlation than show an experiment/intervention changes an outcome.

In my opinion, fail safe N statistics have had their day. Most textbooks about meta-analysis, like Borenstein et al.'s (2021), have moved on to report other statistics (see below); I had to dig out information from Borenstein et al. (2009) to complete this section! In addition, Simonsohn et al. (2014b) argue that researchers may not place entire studies in the file-drawer, instead placing sub-sets of analyses that produce non-significant results, that is, p-hacking. This means estimates of publication bias based on fail-safe n values are unlikely to represent how researchers engage in attempts to overcome a lack of statistical significance. In Chap. 14, I will introduce Simonsohn et al.'s p-curve analysis as a method to account for p-hacking.

Begg and Mazumdar Rank Correlation and Egger's Regression Test

MAJOR outputs two statistics that quantify the relationship between sample size and effect size. Begg and Mazumdar's (1994) Rank correlation test computes the rank correlation between effect size and the standard error, while Egger et al. (1997) proposed a regression test that likewise tests the size of the relationship between effect size and standard error. Both tests are interpreted the same way; a significant result suggests there is a relationship between effect size and standard error, hinting at publication bias. Because larger standard errors indicate smaller sample sizes a positive correlation between standard error and effect size indicates that studies with smaller sample sizes are finding larger effect sizes. I find it useful to consult these statistics when viewing funnel plots.

Funnel Plots

A funnel plot depicts effect size on the x axis and standard error on the y axis for a set of studies included in a meta-analysis. Standard errors represent the amount of dispersion a data point (like an individual effect size) has around the population mean. In meta-analysis, we have effectively generated a population mean by creating a sample-average correlation or effect size difference, so the standard error for each study tells us how much that each effect size differs from the overall effect size. Standard errors are influenced by the sample size; they get smaller the larger the sample size. This is because statistics from a study with a larger sample size are more representative of the population effect size (see Chap. 3), because the sample is closer to the total population sample, and, as a result, this reduces the standard error for studies with larger samples relative to those with smaller samples. In meta-analysis, this plays out in the form of weighting; studies with larger samples are weighted more relative to studies with smaller samples. This means that studies with larger samples necessarily have smaller standard errors relative to the overall effect size—their influence is greater on the overall effect size which means their standard error is smaller compared to studies with less influence/weighting.

A funnel plot can help to identify publication bias because it allows you to see if there is (a) a roughly even number of studies with effect sizes above and below the overall effect size (see Fig. 10.9 for an example of this) and (b) if there are any 'missing' studies, especially at the bottom of the plot where standard errors are greatest (and sample sizes are smallest). In a literature that is not especially affected by publication bias we would expect there to be similar numbers of studies above and below the overall effect size, which is, an average of all the effect sizes we included in the meta-analysis. This does not necessarily mean we should expect that there will be a full range of positive, negative, and null values, because our set of included studies represents a random selection of all possible tests that could be run. As mentioned later in the chapter, meta-analyses of correlations frequently report a range of positive effect sizes, but that does not necessarily mean there is publication bias, just that the range of possible values is bounded, which may reflect limitations in methods used to conduct correlational studies or that there really is a positive relationship between the variables. I would say that it's more likely you'll get a range of positive, negative, and null effect size differences, but even this is not guaranteed and a lack of one kind of effect size does not always indicate publication bias.

A better indicator of publication bias is where you get asymmetry between effect sizes at the bottom of your plot. Recall that the y axis is the standard error of the effect sizes and that studies with smaller sample sizes have larger standard errors. Now if you have a funnel plot where you get a cluster of studies with large standard errors (i.e. small sample sizes) that ALL report positive effects, and your plot lacks an equivalent cluster of studies with large standard errors that ALL report negative (null) effect sizes, then you may have evidence for publication bias. This pattern sounds like publication bias; studies with large, positive effect sizes are published, while studies with smaller positive, negative, or null effect sizes are missing from the published literature. This idea has been taken even further by Uri Simonsohn and colleagues who have created software to run p curve analysis, which specifically looks for studies that have only just reached conventional thresholds of significance, like $p = 0.04$. I'll talk more about this in Chap. 14.

Using Duval and Tweedie's Trim and Fill Method to Adjust the Overall Effect Size for 'Missing Studies'

Imagine that you have a funnel plot which has four studies at the bottom of the funnel plot that are all to the right of the vertical line (the overall effect size). Further imagine that there are no equivalent studies that fall to the left of the vertical line near the bottom of the plot. This pattern, studies with larger positive effects being present, studies with smaller positive (or negative or null effects) being absent, suggests potential publication bias, based on 'missing' studies we would expect if publication bias either did not exist or was less influential in a literature. Duval and Tweedie (2000a, 2000b) proposed a method to adjust the overall effect size for 'missing studies'—the trim and fill method. It's called trim and fill because the method first trims the overall effect size in the same way you can trim a mean by excluding extreme values. This outputs an adjusted estimate of the overall effect size with the extreme values trimmed. The final step of the method is to fill in the 'missing' studies by adding them to the plot. This can be done in several software packages—my experience of using the technique came when using Comprehensive

Meta-Analysis to complete Cooke et al. (2016). You can also see the overall effect size adjusted once the filled studies have been added. However, Simonsohn et al. (2014a) argue that this method has several flaws that make it less effective than p-curve analysis, which we will discuss in Chap. 14.

Ways to Address Publication Bias in a Meta-Analysis

It's one thing to know there is an issue and another to do something about it. In the previous section, I talked a lot about identifying publication bias but not so much about addressing it. One option is to make statistical adjustments to your overall effect size. The Duval and Tweedie missing studies value does that for you. Applying this correction has the effect of adjusting the overall effect size, although it may not change the results too much. While this method is fine for adjusting the effect size after completing a meta-analysis, there are more direct approaches to publication bias that the meta-analyst can take that do not involve statistical corrections. Typically, these take place during your systematic review.

A simple way to address publication bias when running a meta-analysis is to include unpublished results. Unpublished results tend to be called 'grey literature', reflecting a degree of uncertainty about them. Depending on the resources you have available to search for studies, it is well worth considering searching the grey literature. I always tell those I work with on a meta-analysis to check the EThOS database, which is the repository for UK PhD theses. This reflects my experience as a PhD student where I identified one study that was never written up for publication but did appear in an American PhD thesis. It's easy to search EThOS so it's worth considering doing as the standard of work in PhD theses is generally high and there are times when students do not have the time or energy to publish results, especially negative or null results.

Other sources of grey literature include (a) mailshots to memberships of academic bodies, (b) government or charity reports, and (c) the open science framework and pre-print servers. For the last few meta-analyses I've run, I have emailed academic bodies, in my case the Division of Health Psychology, European Health Psychology Society, and UK Society for Behavioural Medicine, to request unpublished findings on the topic I am searching for. Responses to these emails tend to be unpredictable. Sometimes, researchers will send you papers they are working on or that are under review, other times you get nothing in response. Given the limited amount of effort required to send a few emails, it's probably worth doing this if you want to identify unpublished studies.

In my experience, there's not been much point in me including data from government or charity reports when running a meta-analysis. This is not to say that these reports are not useful, just that they rarely report correlations between variables I am interested in or effect size differences in an outcome. Such statistics tend not to be the focus of these reports, which are more likely to report effects over time, like changes in the frequency of people reporting a behaviour, and the reports also often report percentage values that are hard for me to do anything with in a meta-analysis.

Nevertheless, I mention these reports as I know in certain areas important information is reported in this way, so, don't be put off by my experience. If you think you can find useful information then go for it!

Since I started my last meta-analysis, there are now many more unpublished results on the open science framework and psychologists seem to be making more use of pre-print servers like psyarxiv, a repository for unpublished papers. Therefore, it is worth searching these websites for relevant, unpublished data that could be included in your meta-analysis. I'd hazard a guess that there are more negative and null findings on open science resources than you would typically find in journals, so, including relevant results that fit into your meta-analysis topic is a good way to strengthen confidence that your results are not due to publication bias.

Why It's Important to Publish Null and Negative Effect Sizes

I'm going to finish this chapter with an example of the importance of publishing null and negative effect sizes from one of my meta-analyses, Cooke et al. (2016). One of the very best things about meta-analysis is its ability to confound your theories, hunches, and expectations. Prior to running the meta-analyses for Cooke et al. (2016), I'd only ever found positive relationships between variables within the theory of planned behaviour. Although not explicitly mentioned by Ajzen (1991), it seemed to me that we should expect positive relationships between variables and outcomes, and this is what we typically found. For most of my meta-analyses for Cooke et al. (2016), we again found positive relationships between attitudes and intentions, intentions, and behaviour, et cetera. There was one rogue finding where self-efficacy had a negative relationship with drinking intentions, but that was quite easy to explain away as that study had recruited an adolescent sample, most of who were not drinking alcohol yet, so we should perhaps be expecting a negative relationship especially as all the other studies for self-efficacy and intentions reported positive relationships.

However, when it came time to run the forest plots for the relationships between perceived control and intentions and separately perceived control and drinking behaviour, it became apparent that you don't always find positive relationships! Forest plots showed a real mixed-bag of results, including positive, negative, and null correlations. Overall, the sample-weighted average correlations were null, suggesting that perceived control correlated with neither intentions nor drinking behaviour.

Such results presented a challenge to the theory in that we found no evidence for either relationship, which contrasted with other meta-analyses of testing these relationships. Running these analyses made me go back and look at the literature for perceived control and alcohol and it dawned on me that this was not a straightforward relationship. The first paper I read on perceived control and alcohol by Norman et al. (1998) should have alerted me to the idea that a lack of control (i.e. a negative relationship between control and drinking behaviour) can underlie drinking, because that is exactly what Paul and his colleagues said in their paper. There's also a nice paper by Schlegel et al. (1992) which showed that perceived control was an important predictor of drinking among those with an alcohol use disorder, for whom intentions were not significantly associated with drinking, but perceived control did not predict drinking among those without an alcohol use disorder, matching results from our meta-analysis.

Later, I worked with Mark Burgess and Emma Davies looking at results from an open-ended survey of English drinkers (Burgess et al., 2019). Although not specifically focused on control, we found evidence that while many of our sample wanted to remain in control when drinking, a minority reported drinking to get out of control. Of course, one should not get too far ahead of oneself based on results of one study, but it remains the case that without those unusual negative and null findings in the meta-analysis, I might have struggled to explain results in Burgess et al. (2019). Negative and null findings often tell us more than we realise. It's time we valued them more.

Summary

The aim of this chapter was to discuss methods to identify and address publication bias. In the next chapter, I will discuss extensions to meta-analysis to help you develop your knowledge and expertise further.

References

Ajzen, I. (1991). The theory of planned behavior. *Organizational Behavior and Human Decision Processes, 50*, 179–211. https://doi.org/10.1016/0749-5978(91)90020-T

Begg, C. B., & Mazumdar, M. (1994). Operating characteristics of a rank correlation test for publication bias. *Biometrics, 50*, 1088–1101.

Borenstein, M., Hedges, L. V., Higgins, J., & Rothstein, H. R. (Eds.). (2009). *Introduction to meta-analysis* (1st ed.). Wiley.

Borenstein, M., Hedges, L. V., Higgins, J., & Rothstein, H. R. (2021). *Introduction to meta-analysis* (2nd ed.). Wiley.

Burgess, M., Cooke, R., & Davies, E. L. (2019). *My own personal hell*: Approaching and exceeding thresholds of too much alcohol. *Psychology & Health*, 1–19. https://doi.org/10.1080/08870446.2019.1616087

Chambers, C. (2017). *The seven deadly sins of psychology: A manifesto for reforming the culture of scientific practice*. Princeton University Press.

Cooke, R., Dahdah, M., Norman, P., & French, D. P. (2016). How well does the theory of planned behaviour predict alcohol consumption? A systematic review and meta-analysis. *Health Psychology Review, 10*, 148–167. https://doi.org/10.1080/17437199.2014.947547

Duval, S., & Tweedie, R. (2000a). A nonparametric "trim and fill" method of accounting for publication bias in meta-analysis. *Journal of the American Statistical Association, 95*, 89–98.

Duval, S., & Tweedie, R. (2000b). Trim and fill: A simple funnel-plot-based method of testing and adjusting for publication bias in meta-analysis. *Biometrics, 56*, 455–463.

Egger, M., Higgins, J. P. T., & Smith, D. (1997). Bias in meta-analysis detected by a simple, graphical test. *BMJ, 315*, 629–634.

Norman, P., Bennett, P., & Lewis, H. (1998). Understanding binge drinking among young people: An application of the Theory of Planned Behaviour. *Health Education Research, 13*(2), 163–169. https://doi.org/10.1093/her/13.2.163-a

Orwin, R. G. (1983). A fail-safe *N* for effect size in meta-analysis. *Journal of Educational Statistics, 8*(2), 157–159. https://doi.org/10.3102/10769986008002157

Rosenthal, R. R. (1979). The File drawer problem and tolerance for null results. *Psychological Bulletin, 86*, 638–641.

Schlegel, R. P., DAvernas, J. R., Zanna, M. P., DeCourville, N. H., & Manske, S. R. (1992). Problem Drinking: A Problem for the Theory of Reasoned Action?1. *Journal of Applied Social Psychology, 22*(5), 358–385. https://doi.org/10.1111/j.1559-1816.1992.tb01545.x

Simonsohn, U., Nelson, L. D., & Simmons, J. P. (2014a). *p*-curve and effect size: Correcting for publication bias using only significant results. *Perspectives on Psychological Science, 9*(6), 666–681. https://doi.org/10.1177/1745691614553988

Simonsohn, U., Nelson, L. D., & Simmons, J. P. (2014b). P-curve: A key to the file-drawer. *Journal of Experimental Psychology: General, 143*(2), 534–547. https://doi.org/10.1037/a0033242

Further Methods for Meta-Analysis 14

Extensions of Meta-analysis

Having practised conducting meta-analysis in Chaps. 8, 9, and 10 and reflected on issues of meta-analytic method, heterogeneity, and publication bias in Chaps. 11, 12, and 13, you now possess both experience of running meta-analyses and knowledge about what the output of these analyses mean. Of course, like all statistical techniques, there are various extensions of meta-analysis that can be used to embellish your expertise. The aim of this chapter is to introduce some of these extensions, acknowledging that it is beyond the scope of this book to do more than this. I will cover six extensions to meta-analysis: (1) a better way to test publication bias; (2) a special type of moderator analysis; (3) how to estimate the extent of variation of 'true' effect sizes in a random-effects meta-analysis; (4) an alternative method for computing effect size differences that accounts for baseline scores in the outcome; (5) a better method for testing theory relationships using correlational data; and (6) methods to address dependence between multiple outcomes.

Each of these extensions have their own complications and I recommend reading the citations included in each section to build your knowledge. Moreover, only the third extension can easily be done in MAJOR, so, you will need to use other software packages to run these analyses. As stated at the beginning, the goal of this book is to introduce meta-analysis to psychologists, not to tell the whole story. I can only take you so far because I don't know everything. Indeed, I have not conducted many of these extensions myself. Knowing about these extensions is better than not knowing, especially if you end up needing to address these issues in your own meta. A final thing to note about several of these extensions is that the proof of principle papers for some techniques were run on existing meta-analyses. It's great when you can build knowledge of techniques when using already published meta-analyses, which speaks to the broad aim of replication and sharing of knowledge and ideas.

R. Cooke, *Meta-Analysis for Psychologists*,
https://doi.org/10.1007/978-3-031-73773-2_14

A Better Way to Test Publication Bias—p-curve Analysis

In Chap. 13, we covered statistics that can be used to estimate publication bias: Rosenthal and Orwin's Fail-Safe N values, Begg and Mazmuder's Rank Correlation, Egger's regression test and Duval and Tweedie's trim and fill method. Such statistics are commonly reported in meta-analytic papers to inform the reader about the extent of publication bias in studies included in the meta-analysis. However, Simonsohn et al. (2014b) argue that because such statistics only address the issue where non-significant results are put away in the metaphorical file drawer they tell us little about what happens when researchers engage in p-hacking.

Imagine three independent studies on the same topic. Study (a) reports a significant positive effect size where $p = 0.01$, Study (b) reports a positive effect size where $p = 0.06$, not quite meeting the threshold for statistical significance, Study (c) reports a non-significant positive effect size, where $p = 0.40$. Study (a) is most likely to be submitted for publication, while study (c) is probably going to find itself in the file drawer or uploaded to the Open Science Framework. Study (b), however, is at risk of p-hacking because results for the effect size are close to the magic $p < 0.05$, the research team might decide to identify some outliers, whose removal changes the significance level, or collect more data until they get $p < 0.05$. So, the team behind study (b) might end up with sub-sets of data analyses—those that show non-significance are filed, those that show significance are submitted for publication.

Simonsohn et al. argue that p-hacking affects the accuracy of traditional methods of testing for publication bias because research teams may have few 'failed' studies, those showing non-significance, but multiple analyses of these failed studies. So, significant results might not have been significant without p hacking. I believe that psychology is a discipline at high risk of p-hacking because most of the time psychologists complete statistical analyses themselves (see Chap. 6 for a discussion about detection bias).

P-curve analysis can help identify issues of publication bias by assessing the distribution of statistically significant p values for a set of independent findings—like a set of studies included in a meta-analysis. The first thing to draw your attention to is that this analysis does NOT focus on non-significant results. Published, non-significant results are not obvious examples of publication bias! Instead, p-curve analysis looks at the p values for all the significant studies and determines how likely this set of studies suffers from publication bias.

The way p-curve analysis works is breathtakingly simple. When you have a literature without obvious publication bias, you should have a greater number of studies that report more significant results—for example, results where p is 0.01, 0.02, for example. Such results are hard to achieve by p-hacking and more likely represent a true effect. In contrast, a literature containing publication bias, should have multiple studies that report p values close to the threshold of $p < 0.05$, for example, $p = 0.04$, $p = 0.035$. Effect sizes with these levels of significance are more likely to be the result of p-hacking, because it is (relatively) easy to p-hack a result to achieve a p value in this range. This is not to say all results where $p = 0.04$ are the result of p-hacking, just that it is probably easier to achieve a value of $p = 0.04$ by p-hacking relative to a p value of 0.01. P-curve analysis plots the number of p values for a set of studies and outputs results telling you if most of your significant findings have low or high p values.

To run a p-curve analysis based on studies you include in your meta-analysis, you don't need to extract the p values from your primary papers. All you need is the effect size (r, d) and the degrees of freedom. The analysis takes advantage of the degrees of freedom (effectively telling the analysis what the sample size is) to determine the significance of the effect in the time-honoured tradition of looking up a value at the back of your statistics textbook. So, a correlation of $r = 0.89$ will be significant (at $p < 0.05$) with a smaller sample size than a correlation of $r = 0.15$, because the first correlation is much larger than the second one. This follows on from a simple principle that we already know; it's easier to find a significant effect with a larger sample.

At www.p-curve.com there is an app that will let you calculate p-curves. Enter the individual effect sizes from your meta, plus the degrees of freedom (in brackets) and that's it! The output for a set of studies with no evidence of publication bias should be skewed so that most of the p values are near the 0.01, 0.02 end of the x axis, whereas one where there is evidence of publication bias will be skewed so most values are near the 0.04 end of the axis. The output also tells you how many included studies meet $p < 0.05$.

Simonsohn and colleagues have published further papers on p-curve analysis, which I recommend reading if you want to know more. I especially like Simonsohn et al. (2014a) because it shows the limitations of the trim and fill method to identify publication bias, using results from a meta-analysis. Compared to some of the extensions discussed in this chapter, it really is easy to run p-curve analyses following a meta-analysis, so I would encourage you to do so.

A Special Type of Moderator Analysis—meta-CART

Newby et al. (2021) report results of a systematic review and meta-analysis I co-authored with a team of researchers based at Coventry University, led by Dr Katie Newby, Professor Katherine Brown, and Dr Stefanie Williams. The primary goal of the meta-analysis was to estimate the effect of receiving a digital intervention on participants' self-efficacy, that is, their confidence that they can perform a behaviour (Bandura, 1977).

This meta-analysis was broader than meta-analyses that I first author, as we tested the effects of digital interventions aiming to increase self-efficacy across five health behaviours: alcohol consumption, dietary behaviours, physical activity, safe sex, and smoking. The team was keen to see if interventions using different behaviour change techniques, that is, methods to promote behaviour change such as goal-setting, social support, et cetera, were more/less effective at increasing self-efficacy. A further question was if clusters of these techniques, when delivered in the same intervention, would work together to amplify, or attenuate the effects on self-efficacy.

To address this interesting question, Katie invited Xinru Li and Elise Dusseldorp based at Leiden University in the Netherlands to join the team. Xinru and Elise are pioneers in the field of meta-CART (Classification And Regression Trees) who had already published a neat paper where they used data from Susan Michie's meta-analysis on BCTs (Michie et al., 2009) to show the value of meta-CART (Dusseldorp et al., 2014).

Essentially, meta-CART acts as special type of moderator (sub-group) analysis. It seeks to build models that partition studies from a meta-analysis into clusters that cohere, for example, do all the studies that use a particular behaviour change technique, like implementation intentions, have similar effects? It is a form of machine learning that seeks a parsimonious solution to heterogeneity in data. The idea is, can we reduce the heterogeneity in our meta-analysis effect sizes by partitioning studies together? meta-CART is a two-stage process: a classification and regression tree model is built before running a mixed effects meta-analysis (see Chap. 12). The classification aspect of CART reflects categorical factors, whereas the regression aspect covers continuous variables.

We did not find any evidence for clusters of BCTs leading to more or less effective interventions to change self-efficacy in Newby et al. (2021). However, this analysis was based on only 20 studies. A paper by Xinru (Li et al., 2017) clearly showed that meta-CART produced its best results when based on a sample of 120 studies; Michie et al.'s (2009) paper which included over 100 studies. The 20 studies we had were not enough to make the most of this technique. As the number of research studies within a discipline grows, and especially where you have studies reporting results using extremely popular methods like the Behaviour Change Taxonomy, the potential to use meta-CART will increase.

A Method to Estimate Variability Among 'True' Effect Sizes in a Random-Effects Meta-Analysis—Prediction Intervals

Borenstein et al. (2009) note that reporting results from a meta-analysis typically involves focusing on the overall effect size and the confidence intervals about this effect. The overall effect size estimates the magnitude of effect found across included studies while the confidence intervals tell us the precision of this estimate. However, neither statistic tells us how the 'true' effects for each included study are distributed about the overall effect.

When running a fixed-effect meta, this question does not matter because we assume all included studies have the same 'true' effect size which is measured with more or less precision based on sample size. In a random-effects meta-analysis, however, this logic does not hold; recall from Chap. 11 that a random-effects meta-analysis assumes the 'true' effect size might be different for each included study due to a host of factors. A consequence of this assumption is that we need to think about how the true effects are distributed about the overall effect size computed in a meta-analysis. To address this issue, we need to talk about prediction intervals.

A prediction interval is the interval within which a score will fall in a distribution if we select a case at random from the population the distribution is based on. Like confidence intervals, prediction intervals can be calculated with reference to the percentage of the distribution the value should fall within. So, a prediction interval of 95% would mean the value selected would fall in the interval 95% of the time; a 99% interval, the value would fall 99% of the time.

MAJOR allows you to add prediction intervals to the forest plots in your meta-analysis output. Figures 14.1 and 14.2 show the forest plots from Chaps. 9 and 10 with prediction intervals added as lines either side of the diamond at the bottom of the plot. In Fig. 14.1, the prediction intervals range from 0.15 to 0.94 which means 95% of values for the 'true' effect (correlation) between drinking intentions and drinking behaviour across studies will fall between a correlation of $r = 0.15$ and $r = 0.94$. Our overall effect size of $r = 0.55$ is the sample-weighted average based on observations (data) from the ten included studies, with the confidence intervals reflecting error in measurement of this mean. The prediction intervals tell us that we should expect the 'true' effect of drinking intentions on drinking behaviour to fall between $r = 0.15$ and $r = 0.94$, 95% of the time. A few things to note. First, the prediction intervals are both in the same direction (positive), which suggests that most 'true' effects are likely to be positive. Second, the prediction intervals do not include zero which means the 'true' effect is unlikely to be zero in many studies.

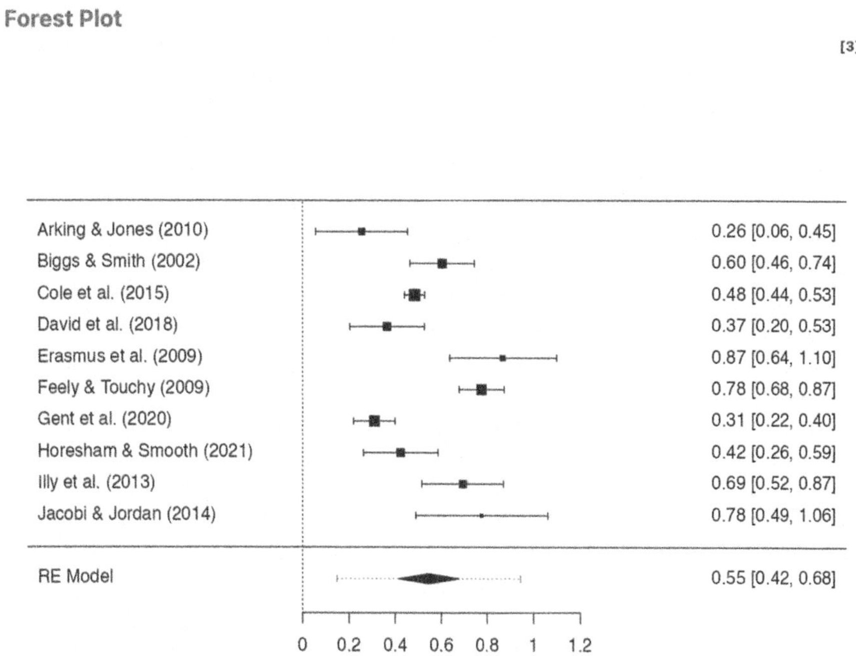

Fig. 14.1 Forest plot for meta-analysis of correlations with prediction intervals

Forest Plot

[3]

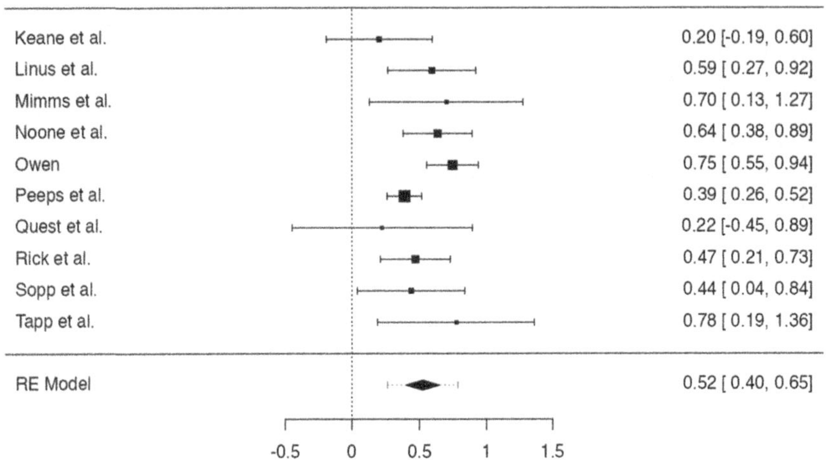

Fig. 14.2 Forest plot for meta-analysis of effect size differences with prediction intervals

In Fig. 14.2, the prediction intervals range from 0.21 to 0.79 which means that 95% of values for the 'true' effect (effect size difference) for screen time for those who received versus did not receive an intervention will fall between $d = 0.21$ and $d = 0.79$. Our overall effect size of $d = 0.52$ is the sample-weighted average based on observations (data) from the ten included studies, with the confidence intervals reflecting error in measurement of the mean. The prediction intervals tell us that we should expect the 'true' effect of drinking intentions on drinking behaviour to fall between $d = 0.21$ and $d = 0.79$, 95% of the time. As both prediction intervals are in the same direction (positive) we should expect most 'true' effects to find positive effect size differences, rather than negative or null effects.

In addition, because the intervals do not include zero, the 'true' effect is unlikely to be zero in many studies.

Confidence intervals reflect error in measurement of the mean. In meta-analysis, an overall effect size's error in measurement is strongly tied to the number of studies you include. If you have five studies, then you are likely to have wider confidence intervals than if you have 50, or 500 studies looking at the same effect size. So, the more studies you include in your meta, the narrower the confidence intervals for the overall effect size. By contrast, prediction intervals reflect both error in measurement of the mean, which is affected by the number of studies, and variance in the studies, represented by Tau^2, which is not affected by the number of studies. So, three meta-analyses containing five, 50 or 500 studies of the same effect size will have similar prediction interval's because Tau^2 is not sensitive to the number of studies included in the meta-analysis, whereas their confidence intervals will inevitably be narrower in the set of 500 studies than the set of 50 or 5 studies. In sum, the prediction interval is telling you the range of possible values the 'true' effect sizes could take, under the assumption that the 'true' effect size for each study might differ. Despite being under-reported, prediction intervals should be reported routinely given that most papers report results of random-effects meta-analyses and therefore we need to be able to see the range of 'true' effects we expect there to be based on the effect sizes we enter in our meta. The fact that it is easy to add prediction intervals to your forest plot also counts in their favour.

A Method to Control for Baseline Differences in an Outcome Prior to Running a Meta-Analysis of Effect Size Differences

The typical approach taken in a meta-analysis of effect size differences is to compute the overall effect size difference in the outcome(s) for two groups at follow-up. In an RCT, this is a reasonable approach to take; clinical trials units that run RCTs do all they can to ensure participants in each group do not differ greatly in their baseline outcome scores. So, it makes sense to look only for between group differences in outcome scores at follow-up, that is, when sufficient time has passed for the intervention to have shown some effect on the outcome.

In contrast, psychology studies are not always run under such strict conditions, which means that controlling for baseline differences in an outcome might be advisable or even necessary. Imagine your two groups' scores in screen time intervention study are as indicated in Table 14.1.

Looking at the follow-up column, it appears our intervention has successfully reduced screen time, with a large-sized d value of 0.96. However, if we look at the baseline column, there's an even bigger difference between the two groups: $d = 2.01$. Unlike in an RCT, the two groups' baseline scores on the outcome are obviously different, with control scores larger than intervention scores.

Why does this matter? Well, if we only meta-analyse the results from follow-up, we might end up with a more positive (or negative) view of what is happening in this study. Our initial comparison at follow-up suggests a positive effect size, indicating a benefit of receiving the intervention. But is that what's really happening, or is there another explanation?

I first started thinking about this issue after I was asked about controlling for baseline differences in alcohol outcomes at a conference where I was presenting preliminary results for what became Cooke et al. (2023). I worked with my

Table 14.1 Control and intervention groups' screen time scores at baseline and follow-up

Condition	Baseline (M, SD)	Follow-up (M, SD)
Control	30.00 (5.45)	20.00 (5.15)
Intervention	20.00 (4.45)	15.00 (5.25)
d (between groups)	2.01	0.96

co-author Paul Norman on this issue. Paul had come across a paper by Morris (2008) which directly addressed the issue of baseline corrections in effect sizes. In essence, what you do is generate mean difference values for each group, by subtracting the baseline from the follow-up, subtract these values from one another before dividing the result by the pooled standard deviation using baseline values. Morris argues that assuming your intervention works, you should expect greater variance in scores at follow-up than baseline (where you are assuming groups are more similar in their scores) and goes on to demonstrate in his paper that dividing mean values by baseline (pre-test) standard deviations is justified to generate your effect size difference.

I must acknowledge there are challenges involved in running a meta-analysis of effect size differences adopting Morris' approach. Using Morris' formula meant I had to go through an extra step of re-calculating effect size differences before running the meta-analysis and the method had other disadvantages, including exclusion of papers from meta-analysis that had not reported baseline statistics for each group. Unless you have statistics for both timepoints, you cannot run this analysis. There's also the question of whether the extra effort is justified. As mentioned above, if the studies you are meta-analysing use high-quality study designs, and do not show obvious differences between groups in baseline scores, it may not be appropriate to run meta-analysis this way. Nevertheless, I report this method here as I've used it, and it may be valuable for others to use it too.

A Better Method for Testing Theory Relationships Using Correlational Data

One of the first workshops I ran on meta-analysis threw up a good question—'What happens if you wanted to meta-analyse regression coefficients?' A key limitation of correlations, and therefore also meta-analyses of correlations, is that a correlation between two variables does not control for the effects of other variables, which means you cannot be sure that the effect sizes you are pooling would not remain unaffected by inclusion of additional variables. We know correlations are limited from an inference standpoint; that's why we teach psychology students to run regression analyses!

It took me a while to appreciate the importance of this question and the penny only really dropped when I read Martin Hagger's paper (Hagger et al., 2016) showing the way to run a meta-analysis of coefficients from regression models. Martin and his colleagues had reanalysed the data from Cooke et al. (2016) and McDermott et al. (2015), who reported a meta-analysis of correlations testing theory of planned behaviour relationships for dietary behaviours, to provide examples of a better method for testing theory relationships using correlations.

The goal was to provide a 'simultaneous omnibus test of the theory…to adequately test theory predictions' (p. 8). They estimated a path analysis based on an 'augmented matrix of meta-analytically derived correlations' (p. 8). The first step was to conduct additional data extraction from the papers included in the two metas, extracting the intercorrelations between the predictors of intentions, that is, the correlations between attitudes and subjective norms, between attitudes and perceived behaviour control; subjective norms and perceived behavioural control. Each of these correlations was extracted from the included studies in each of the original meta-analyses, before being pooled using random effects meta-analysis into r_+. The values they generated are reported in Table 1 of the paper. Table 2 contains both these correlations plus the ones already reported in the original meta-analyses, that is, the attitude-intention correlation of $r_+ = 0.62$ from Cooke et al. (2016) is reported.

The next step Martin and colleagues took was to input these values into path-analytic models in MPlus for each meta-analysis, which they report in Table 3 of their paper. At first glance, not much seems to have changed from the original meta-analyses; in Cooke et al. (2016) we found evidence for significant attitude–intention, subjective norm intention, and intention–behaviour relationships, and limited evidence that perceived behavioural control was associated with drinking behaviour.

The key difference is the *statistic* that's being reported for each theory relationship, a beta value, like you get in a multiple regression. These statistics are showing the effects of attitudes on intention while simultaneously accounting for the effects of subjective norms, and perceived behavioural control. Doing this increases confidence in results. In Cooke et al. (2016), we reported a sample-weighted average correlation between attitudes and intentions of $r_+ = 0.62$. In Hagger et al. (2016), attitudes are shown, across studies, to significantly *predict* intentions beta = 0.51. So, even when the effects of other predictors, subjective norms, perceived behavioural control, are included in a regression model, attitudes remain significant predictors of drinking intentions. This approach allows research teams to run secondary analyses in the same way as we would if we were analysing a primary dataset, which is an excellent development.

One of the few downsides of the approach reported in Hagger et al. (2016) is that path analyses were run using MPlus, which, as a licensed software package, may not be accessible. Happily, alternative methods for running path analyses are now possible in R, including the MASEM method (Cheung & Hong, 2017), so path analysis within meta-analysis is available to all.

As I have not yet run such analyses myself, I am reluctant to go further than to recommend it when testing theory relationships in psychology. Martin has published several papers using these methods since the one I discussed, including his updated meta-analysis (Hagger et al., 2017) of the common-sense model of illness and a recent meta-analysis of studies testing theory of planned behaviour relationships using longitudinal designs (Hagger & Hamilton, 2023). I recommend reading these papers to increase your knowledge further.

Methods to Address Dependence Between Multiple Outcomes

An important, but often overlooked, issue in meta-analysis is the need for effect sizes to be independent of one another (see Chap. 7). Part of conducting a meta-analysis is to ensure that each effect size you pool does not represent data from any other effect size you include and to take care when including multiple measures of an effect size within the same analysis. Where effect sizes have dependency, by being related to one another, including both in a meta of ostensibly independent effect sizes is like double-counting results in an election, adding greater weight to certain effects relative to others.

In each of the meta-analyses I have authored, I had to address issues of dependency between measures, with one or more of the following occurring: (1) papers reporting multiple studies based on recruitment of independent samples; (2) papers reporting effect sizes for sub-samples; (3) papers reporting effect sizes for multiple timepoints. For (1), we argued that these datasets were independent of each other; the authors reported them as Study 1, Study 2, Study 3, and it was not obvious that participants from any sample took part in more than one study. When extracting data, be careful, as this can happen—one of my papers (Cooke & Sheeran, 2013) reports three studies, the first based on the total sample we recruited, and the other two based on sub-samples recruited from within the original sample. For (2) we treated the sub-samples (e.g. effect sizes for men and women reported separately) as independent. One issue with this approach is that when you pool results across all studies, your samples lack comparability; correlations based on a sample of female and male students might be different to correlations based on just male or just female students. Indeed, we found some evidence to support this claim (see discussion in Cooke et al., 2016).

For (3), the response is more challenging. In Cooke and French (2008), we had papers where the correlation between variables was reported on multiple occasions using a longitudinal design. Our options were to either include correlations for all timepoints and use each sample size or the average of the correlations and choose between the sample sizes. We opted for the second option, because we felt that the first option is a clear example of dependence in results. If I have a paper that reports effect sizes from samples that contain at least some of the same participants, it is likely that these correlations will correlate with one another as people tend to be consistent when answering survey measures.

Martin Hagger's (2022) paper offers some excellent advice on how to address dependence in meta-analysis. Martin argues against aggregation of effect sizes from the same sample due to the likelihood that this will inflate effects. So, what I did in Cooke and Sheeran (2004) is not recommended! I'd argue that what we did in Cooke and French (2008), where we averaged effect sizes from multiple timepoints into one effect size and used the smallest sample available, is less problematic. While I believe this is better than including the effect size for each timepoint, which are likely to be dependent, you are still reducing the power of your analysis by using the smallest sample size. Martin discusses two alternative methods to deal with dependency: multi-level meta-analysis and robust variance estimation.

The multi-level approach partitions variance into three components (1) sampling error (see Chap. 11); (2) variability due to multiple effect sizes from the same study; (3) variability due to effects from different studies. So, (2) directly addresses the issue of dependence, modelling the effect sizes for multiple effect sizes from the same study and correcting for variance. Robust variance estimation (Hedges et al. 2010) approximates the average effect size from a set of studies from the same lab/research team, by applying a 'working model' of the dependence structure among effects in included studies. You can run both methods at the same time as they address different aspects of dependence.

While I have yet to use either of these methods, I think robust variance estimation would better suit my needs as I prefer not to include multiple measures of the same outcome within the same meta-analysis but I often include studies from the same research team or laboratory. If you do want to include multiple effect sizes from the same paper, the multi-level approach sounds like the best approach to take. Further details can be found in Gucciardi et al. (Gucciardi et al., 2022).

Summary

The aim of this chapter was to introduce some extensions of meta-analysis. I do not expect you to adopt all these techniques within your own meta-analysis but would recommend you report prediction intervals with your results and consider running a p-curve analysis of your effect sizes. Both are low-cost additions to your meta-analysis paper that will improve its quality. Using other approaches, especially meta-CART, depend on the number of studies you have, and I appreciate you may not wish to dive headlong into running meta-level modelling or path analysis. Ultimately, you may find that these approaches help answer your questions in greater depth and that is why they are included. The final chapter of the book provides advice about how to write up results of your meta-analysis for submission to a peer-review journal.

References

Bandura, A. (1977). Self-efficacy: Toward a unifying theory of behavioral change. *Psychological Review, 84*(2), 191–215.

Borenstein, M., Hedges, L. V., Higgins, J., & Rothstein, H. R. (Eds.). (2009). *Introduction to meta-analysis* (1st ed.). Wiley.

Cheung, M. W.-L., & Hong, R. Y. (2017). Applications of meta-analytic structural equation modelling in health psychology: Examples, issues, and recommendations. *Health Psychology Review, 11*(3), 265–279. https://doi.org/10.1080/17437199.2017.1343678

Cooke, R., Dahdah, M., Norman, P., & French, D. P. (2016). How well does the theory of planned behaviour predict alcohol consumption? A systematic review and meta-analysis. *Health Psychology Review, 10*, 148–167. https://doi.org/10.1080/17437199.2014.947547

Cooke, R., & French, D. P. (2008). How well do the theory of reasoned action and theory of planned behaviour predict intentions and attendance at screening programmes? A meta-analysis. *Psychology & Health, 23*(7), 745–765. https://doi.org/10.1080/08870440701544437

Cooke, R., McEwan, H., & Norman, P. (2023). The effect of forming implementation intentions on alcohol consumption: A systematic review and meta-analysis. *Drug and Alcohol Review, 42*, 68–80. https://doi.org/10.1111/dar.13553

Cooke, R., & Sheeran, P. (2004). Moderation of cognition-intention and cognition-behaviour relations: A meta-analysis of properties of variables from the theory of planned behaviour. *The British Journal of Social Psychology, 43*(Pt 2), 159–186. https://doi.org/10.1348/0144666041501688

Cooke, R., & Sheeran, P. (2013). Properties of intention: Component structure and consequences for behavior, information processing, and resistance. *Journal of Applied Social Psychology, 43*(4), 749–760. https://doi.org/10.1111/jasp.12003

Dusseldorp, E., Van Genugten, L., Van Buuren, S., Verheijden, M. W., & Van Empelen, P. (2014). Combinations of techniques that effectively change health behavior: Evidence from Meta-CART analysis. *Health Psychology, 33*(12), 1530–1540. https://doi.org/10.1037/hea0000018

Gucciardi, D. F., Lines, R. L. J., & Ntoumanis, N. (2022). Handling effect size dependency in meta-analysis. *International Review of Sport and Exercise Psychology, 15*(1), 152–178. https://doi.org/10.1080/1750984X.2021.1946835

Hagger, M. S. (2022). Meta-analysis. *International Review of Sport and Exercise Psychology, 15*(1), 120–151. https://doi.org/10.1080/1750984X.2021.1966824

Hedges, L.V., Tipton, E., Johnson, M.C (2010). Robust variance estimation in meta regression with dependent effect size estimates. *Research Synthesis Methods, 1*(1), 39-65. https://doi.org/10.1080/10.1002/jrsm5

Hagger, M. S., Chan, D. K. C., Protogerou, C., & Chatzisarantis, N. L. D. (2016). Using meta-analytic path analysis to test theoretical predictions in health behavior: An illustration based on meta-analyses of the theory of planned behavior. *Preventive Medicine, 89*, 154–161. https://doi.org/10.1016/j.ypmed.2016.05.020

Hagger, M. S., & Hamilton, K. (2023). Longitudinal tests of the theory of planned behaviour: A meta-analysis. *European Review of Social Psychology*, 1–57. https://doi.org/10.1080/10463283.2023.2225897

Hagger, M. S., Koch, S., Chatzisarantis, N. L. D., & Orbell, S. (2017). The common sense model of self-regulation: Meta-analysis and test of a process model. *Psychological Bulletin, 143*(11), 1117–1154. https://doi.org/10.1037/bul0000118

Li, X., Dusseldorp, E., & Meulman, J. J. (2017). Meta-CART: A tool to identify interactions between moderators in meta-analysis. *British Journal of Mathematical and Statistical Psychology, 70*(1), 118–136. https://doi.org/10.1111/bmsp.12088

McDermott, M., Oliver, M., Simnadis, T., Beck, E. J., Coltman, T., Iverson, D., Caputi, P., & Sharma, R. (2015). The theory of planned behaviour and dietary patterns: A systematic review and meta-analysis. *Preventive Medicine, 81*, 150–156.

Michie, S., Abraham, C., Whittington, C., McAteer, J., & Gupta, S. (2009). Effective techniques in healthy eating and physical activity interventions: A meta-regression. *Health Psychology, 28*(6), 690–701. https://doi.org/10.1037/a0016136

Morris, S. B. (2008). Estimating effect sizes from pretest-posttest-control group designs. *Organizational Research Methods, 11*(2), 364–386. https://doi.org/10.1177/1094428106291059

Newby, K., Teah, G., Cooke, R., Li, X., Brown, K., Salisbury-Finch, B., Kwah, K., Bartle, N., Curtis, K., Fulton, E., Parsons, J., Dusseldorp, E., & Williams, S. L. (2021). Do automated digital health behaviour change interventions have a positive effect on self-efficacy? A systematic review and meta-analysis. *Health Psychology Review, 15*(1), 140–158. https://doi.org/10.1080/17437199.2019.1705873

Simonsohn, U., Nelson, L. D., & Simmons, J. P. (2014a). *p*-curve and effect size: Correcting for publication bias using only significant results. *Perspectives on Psychological Science, 9*(6), 666–681. https://doi.org/10.1177/1745691614553988

Simonsohn, U., Nelson, L. D., & Simmons, J. P. (2014b). *p*-curve: A key to the file-drawer. *Journal of Experimental Psychology: General, 143*(2), 534–547. https://doi.org/10.1037/a0033242

Writing Up Your Meta-Analysis 15

Writing Up Your Meta-Analysis

My academic training is unusual in that the first thing I did during my PhD was conduct a meta-analysis, which became my first publication (Cooke & Sheeran, 2004). It was a steep learning curve, but I received lots of help from my supervisor, Prof Paschal Sheeran, and was supported by other PhD students conducting their own meta-analyses. In many ways, it was the best environment to learn how to write up a meta-analysis.

Much of what you need to write in a meta-analysis paper is the same as what is required for other papers that report the results of quantitative analyses. The main sections, an introduction that sets the scene for the study, a method that details what was done, a results section outlining what was found, and a discussion that summarises what was found, how results compare to other studies and points the way for future research, are all included in a meta-analytic paper. Where things differ is what appears in each of those sections. Sometimes material is a slightly modified form of what is required in a primary paper, other times, you report completely different material. I'll go through each section of the paper with some hints and tips to help you out when you're writing up your meta.

Sections of an Academic Paper

Title Page

I recommend you include the phrase meta-analysis in your title.

R. Cooke, *Meta-Analysis for Psychologists*,
https://doi.org/10.1007/978-3-031-73773-2_15

Abstract

A meta-analysis abstract is a little different to the abstract reporting results from a primary study. Rather than a research question, include a review question, to make it obvious that you are reporting results of a review. The method section should outline some details of the meta-analysis, including the number of studies and the search engines you searched. You might mention running a random effects (or fixed effect) meta-analysis and maybe mention the software you used. Depends a bit on word count. One thing you should do is to report the key statistics your meta-analysis has generated, for example, the sample-weighted average correlation(s) (r_+) or the sample weighted average effect size difference(s) (d_+) and the confidence intervals for these statistics. These are your main findings—the equivalent of saying how much variance your regression model accounted for other the difference between conditions in an ANOVA and need to be highlighted in the abstract. I like to report if moderator variables affect results, but typically do this in less detail due to word count. I recommend ending with conclusions about what the results tell us.

Introduction

An important difference with the introduction of a meta-analysis and the introduction of a primary paper relates to what you are going to do in this section after the opening paragraph. In a primary paper, you often follow your opening paragraph about the main topic of interest (drinking behaviour, illness, screen time, etc.) with a review of the literature, which provides a rationale for what you did in your study. In contrast, in the introduction section of a meta-analysis, you don't want to do too much of this because the results of your study are a literature review! Spending a page and a half of text reviewing the literature seems redundant when the results section is going to do that. So, I always advise those working on meta-analysis to try and limit the literature review to the essentials; it's obvious in a review paper that you need some reference to past literature, but don't overdo it. As my meta-analyses often test theoretical predictions, you can summarise what previous results tell us regarding theory. This will help with your rationale. Alternatively, you can discuss intervention approaches, such as methods or models to inform interventions, or how interventions are delivered and developed, if you are synthesising an intervention literature, or experimental metho ds if pooling experimental manipulations.

Another difference between primary papers and meta-analytic papers is about how you frame the rationale for the review that informs the meta-analysis. Paschal taught me to provide a clear rationale for why the review is needed. You can easily identify these sections in my meta-analyses as they relate to limitations with previous metas. Here're two examples:

- In Cooke et al. (2016), we had to justify why a meta-analysis of theory of planned behaviour alcohol studies was needed, given McEachan et al.'s (2011) excellent meta-analysis of health behaviours based on this theory was already published.

We argued that a limitation of McEachan et al.'s review was that they synthesised results across substance use behaviours (alcohol, drug use, smoking) meaning their results did not give a precise estimate of the magnitude of relationships for alcohol studies. We further argued that because they only found five studies on alcohol, while we had found 33 predicting drinking intentions, we could summarise a wider literature.

- In Cooke et al. (2023), Malaguti et al.'s (2020) meta-analysis of implementation intentions and substance use (alcohol, smoking) studies had been published. We had to justify what our meta-analysis would add to the literature which we did by noting limitations of their meta-analysis, for example, that they had pooled effect size differences across alcohol outcomes (weekly drinking and binge drinking), which we argued meant that it was impossible to precisely determine effect sizes for either outcome.

In both cases, we argued that our meta would provide a more precise estimate of effect sizes. The final thing to say about the Introduction is to always report your review questions at the end of the section, like you would with your hypotheses or research questions in a primary study. I like to have overall review questions and moderator questions. This idea comes from Sheeran and Orbell (1998). If it ain't broke don't fix it.

Method

The method section of a meta-analysis clearly diverges from the method section of a primary paper reporting quantitative designs. This is obvious from the sub-sections, which have different titles to the ones used in primary papers. For instance, we talk about studies rather than participant characteristics, and report results of a systematic review that informed the meta-analysis which is not often done in primary papers. This is a consequence of reporting results of a secondary analysis based on more than one dataset. I'll talk through the sub-sections I've used in the meta-analyses I've published to illustrate key differences.

Search Strategy and Inclusion Criteria

In all my metas, I have always had a sub-section in the method that covered how I found relevant studies and the inclusion criteria, though it should be acknowledged that the name I have used for this section has changed over time. Another thing that has changed from Cooke and Sheeran (2004) to Cooke et al. (2023) is that this sub-section has moved from a meta-analysis format to embrace a systematic review format, where I describe how the review was conducted in greater depth. The aim is for transparent and replicable reporting. One way to do this is to pre-register your review on PROSPERO (or Open Science Framework) and follow PRISMA reporting guidelines. I've used the latter since Cooke et al. (2016) and the former in Cooke et al. (2023). I recommend you do both in your meta-analysis. Within this sub-section of the method, I often have sub-sub-sections describing different parts of what was done.

Search strategy. I have used similar search strategies in all four of my meta-analyses; I've always searched bibliographic databases using search terms and I've also searched reference lists of included studies. In all papers, I've also sent emails requesting unpublished or in-press papers on the review topic. In most of my metas, this involved emailing authors of included studies to request other data they had, following the assumption that if they have already published a relevant paper, they may have other data that I could potentially include in my meta. A limitation with this approach is that does not allow you to find unpublished studies by authors who are yet to publish on the review topic. So, in Cooke et al. (2023), we adopted a different approach where we emailed mailing lists of societies I am a member of: Division of Health Psychology, European Health Psychology, UK Society for Behavioural Medicine, to try and reach a wider audience. It's worth noting that emailing anyone, either directly following publication of a relevant paper, or a mailing list, introduces bias into your search because there is no guarantee that your email will be responded to in the same way that someone else's email is responded to. This contrasts with searching databases and reference lists, which should be replicable by an independent review team.

Inclusion criteria. Inclusion criteria for my four meta-analyses are alike. Most include a criterion about results being published in English, and they all explicitly mention an effect size, or statistics needed to calculate an effect size; in a meta, you should be specifying an inclusion criterion about statistical information to ensure included studies can be pooled. Other criteria varied depending on the topic: Cooke and French (2008) mentions screening; Cooke et al. (2016) drinking behaviour; Cooke et al. (2023) weekly alcohol consumption and/or heavy episodic drinking. All bar Cooke et al. (2023) mentioned theory relationships, whereas Cooke et al. (2023) mentioned groups being asked to form or not implementation intentions.

Selection of studies. Cooke and Sheeran (2004) and Cooke and French (2008) were the result of me searching and screening papers on my own. In contrast, Cooke et al. (2016) and Cooke et al. (2023) involved me and another reviewer (Mary Dahdah in the former paper, Helen McEwan in the latter paper) independently searching and screening papers. This necessitated adding a 'Selection of Studies' sub-section in these papers to detail this process. I'd recommend you follow best practice in searching and screening by involving at least one other independent person to check your selection of studies (see Chap. 4).

Assessment of methodological quality. Cooke et al. (2023) was the first time I reported quality assessment of the studies included in a meta-analysis. We used the Cochrane Risk of Bias tool and provided some detail about this.

Data extraction and coding. In both Cooke et al. (2016) and Cooke et al. (2023), two authors independently extracted the data, which is best practice in systematic reviewing. Both papers involved coding papers too. In Cooke et al. (2023), this involved coding papers for moderator analyses. Things were a bit more complex in Cooke et al. (2016). First, Paul Norman (the third author) and I independently coded the items used to assess perceived behavioural control, self-efficacy, and perceived control as there was lots of heterogeneity in how these constructs were measured in included studies. Second, we spotted that there were 20 different definitions of alcohol consumption in 44 papers included in one or more of the meta-analyses! David French (the fourth author) and I coded the 20 definitions into clusters representing similar phenomena. We ended up with five categories representing different drinking patterns: Getting drunk; Heavy Episodic Drinking; Light Episodic drinking; Quantity of Drinks Consumed; Not Drinking. Having coded the studies in this way, we used this newly created coding frame as a basis for moderation analyses for our studies. Based on my experience, most of the time you'll be coding papers for moderator analyses, rather than coming up with an entirely new categorisation scheme.

Meta-Analytic Strategy (Data Synthesis)

When writing up results of a meta-analysis, it is critical to specify how you calculated your overall effect size. Table 15.1 summarises how I did this in the four meta-analyses I first-authored. In both Cooke and Sheeran (2004) and Cooke and French (2008), I reported calculating the weighted average of correlations, r_+, using a r-to-z transform. In this method, you turn each correlation (r) into a Z score, use the Z scores to calculate the overall effect size, before converting the overall Z score back into an r value to give you r_+. Although it does not say it in either paper, we used the Schmidt-Hunter method, which is a random-effects method. Both papers also contained details on how we assessed homogeneity of effect sizes using the chi-square statistic (Hunter et al., 1982), as well as noting that analyses were run in Schwarzer's

Table 15.1 Summary of meta-analytic strategies I've used

Paper	Meta-analytic method	Software	Heterogeneity test(s)	Publication bias
Cooke and Sheeran (2004)	Schmidt-Hunter	META	Chi-square (Q)	Fail-Safe N
Cooke and French (2008)	Schmidt-Hunter	META	Chi-square (Q)	Fail-Safe N
Cooke et al. (2016)	DerSimonian-Laird	Comprehensive Meta-Analysis	Chi-square (Q); I^2	Fail-Safe N; Duval & Tweedie Trim & Fill
Cooke et al. (2023)	Restricted Maximum Likelihood	metafor	Chi-square (Q); I^2	Fail-Safe N; Egger's regression test

(Schwarzer, 1988) *Meta* computer program. Two further details were included in Cooke and French (2008). First, I mentioned including Fail-Safe N values (Rosenthal, 1979). Second, I explicitly mentioned Cohen's (1992) guidelines for interpretation of magnitude of correlations (see Chap. 3). I did the same in Cooke et al. (2016) and reported guidelines for effect size differences in Cooke et al. (2023).

By the time we get to Cooke et al. (2016), I had moved on to Comprehensive Meta Analysis (Borenstein et al., 2005) and explicitly mention running a random effects meta-analysis. Other changes include referencing forest and funnel plots. There's an indirect reference to the fact that we had categorical moderator variables because I mention doing paired Z tests, and a more explicit mention of Publication bias using funnel plots and Duval and Tweedie's trim and fill method.

In Cooke et al. (2023), I noted that we used Morris' (2008) recommendations to control for baseline differences when we calculated effect size differences (see Chap. 14). I used the metafor package to run meta-analyses in R, which is the software MAJOR runs in jamovi. There's also text about how we calculated effect size differences so that negative values indicated greater reduction in alcohol consumption/heavy episodic drinking by the intervention group (see Chap. 7). There's greater detail on publication bias statistics and more information on both homogeneity statistics, with I^2 mentioned, and more detailed explanation of how we tested moderators using meta regression and mixed effects meta-analysis (see Chap. 12).

Multiple Samples and Multiple Measures

In all my meta-analyses, I've included a sub-section detailing with issues of dependence in effect sizes, that is, how we've dealt with multiple samples coming from the same paper and similar issues. This happened in Cooke and Sheeran (2004) and every meta since has had some variant of this issue. As discussed in greater depth in Chap. 14, there are statistical methods to address dependence among effect sizes, so, I'll end this section by noting that it is possible you will face this issue, so this sub-section is where you outline the approach you decided to take.

Results

Like the method section, the results section for a meta-analytic paper is different to the results section for a primary paper. These are the sub-sections I have used in results sections of my meta-analyses.

Study Characteristics

In both Cooke et al. (2016) and Cooke et al. (2023), I included a Study Characteristics sub-section. I use this sub-section to outline key information about the included studies, akin to describing the sample's characteristics in a primary paper. Like primary papers, I do my best to summarise the gender distribution, the age range (or average age), and sample type (e.g. university student, community) of samples reported in included studies.

However, one thing I've learned doing data extraction for meta-analyses is that reporting of basic study details, like the numbers of men and women in the sample, average age of sample, varies between studies. For example, when coding studies during data extraction for Cooke et al. (2016), I wanted to include the average age of the sample for each study. After coding the first five papers, only one of them had reported the average age of their sample. I then got to my paper (Cooke & French, 2011) and realised I had not reported the average age of my sample either! By the end of data extraction, I'd learned that while most of the studies did report their sample(s) average age, this information was not always reported.

Additional information about studies that's useful to report in a meta-analysis includes (a) country of recruitment; (b) study sample sizes; (c) publication year and (d) total number of studies included and the total number of samples. Reporting information about country of recruitment can help with interpretation later in the paper. For instance, in both Cooke et al. (2016) and Cooke et al. (2023), most included studies were conducted in the UK. This means you need to be careful about generalising results to other countries. Alternatively, the range of sample sizes reported by included studies allows you to consider the power of the studies. Publication year might be useful to discuss if there has been a change in a definition or policy in your literature.

The total number of studies is probably the most important information to report because it tells you a lot about the literature you are meta-analysing. In Cooke et al. (2016), we included 28 *papers* reporting 40 *studies*. It's quite common in meta-analysis to include results from a paper that reports multiple studies. For example, we included three studies from Conner et al. (1999) in Cooke et al. (2016). As these were independent samples, this is fine, although it does mean that you trip over sometimes when talking about the number of effect sizes you include as it's the number of samples rather than the number of papers. I've moved away from papers to talking about samples because there are times when the same paper includes one study with multiple samples. In Cooke et al. (2023), we included multiple, independent, samples from Norman et al. (2018). This study used a fully factorial design with three factors, creating eight independent samples. Initially, we extracted the control condition (who received none of the three interventions) and the group that only received the implementation intention intervention (and neither of the other two). Following discussion, we realised that we could include further comparisons between groups that received the same interventions but either did or did not form implementation intentions. This increased the number of samples we could meta-analyse. It's important to report this information in your results section.

Main Effects

You should always report the main or overall effect size and the confidence intervals from your meta-analysis. You may have quite a few of these, so, put them in a table and describe sparingly to save word count. Nevertheless, it is important to report results across all (or most) included studies as it provides a framework for the remainder of the results section. In Cooke and French (2008), I was pushed for word count so did not report the results for the five theories of planned behaviour relationships in the main body of the text, instead, putting the statistics in a table. In hindsight, I think this is a mistake and in Cooke et al. (2016), where there were nine relationships, I still found space to report each overall effect size. This was particularly important as the overall effect sizes varied considerably from one another with three null relationships being worthy of highlighting. Refer to forest plots in this section to help readers see the dispersion of effect sizes across included studies. In Cooke et al. (2023), the main effect section is split into two paragraphs because we were meta-analysing two outcomes (weekly drinking, heavy episodic drinking). This split also occurred because there was a positive effect for weekly drinking and a null effect for heavy episodic drinking. If both effect sizes had been of similar direction (i.e. both null, both positive, both negative) I might have put them in the same paragraph.

Other statistics to report in the main effects section relate to heterogeneity (see Chap. 12) and publication bias (see Chap. 13). In my meta-analyses to date, there's a general pattern of me finding heterogeneity in overall effect sizes, which leads into a discussion of moderators (see next section). I've generally found a lack of evidence of publication bias, although in Cooke et al. (2016), we did find evidence of publication bias for two relationships (perceived behavioural control-intentions; self-efficacy-intentions). Closer inspection of the self-efficacy–intention relationship using a sensitivity analysis suggested that publication bias for this relationship was an artefact of including results from a study with a different sample age to all other included studies. We were more convinced that there was publication bias for the perceived control–intention relationship so reported the effect size as well as the adjusted effect size following the Trim and Fill method (see Chap. 13). You can also include funnel plots to comment on the presence or absence of publication bias.

Moderator Analyses

I've included moderator analyses in all my meta-analyses. I've looked at factors like publication status (published vs unpublished; Cooke & Sheeran, 2004), time between measurement/length of follow-up (Cooke et al., 2023; Cooke & Sheeran, 2004), type of screening test (Cooke & French, 2008), location of recruitment (i.e. were participants recruited in response to a letter from their GP, a screening service; Cooke & French, 2008), cost of screening (Cooke & French, 2008), whether participants were sent an invitation to screen (Cooke & French, 2008), pattern of consumption (Cooke et al., 2016), gender distribution (Cooke et al., 2016), age of participants (Cooke et al., 2016), sample type (i.e. university vs community, Cooke et al., 2023), mode of delivery (i.e. paper vs online, Cooke et al., 2023), intervention format (i.e. type of implementation intention, Cooke et al., 2023).

There are two takeaway messages from this list. First, there's little consistency in the moderators we tested across the metas. This reflects the idea that moderator analyses tend to be specific to the meta-analysis you are conducting. Experimental factors, like intervention type, are unlikely to be relevant for meta-analyses of correlations. Behaviour-specific moderators, like those focused on screening type, or pattern of consumption, are only relevant if your meta-analysis focuses on those behaviours. Second, that we included moderator analyses in all four meta papers tells you that in each paper, there was heterogeneity in overall effect sizes. This was true of both meta-analysis of correlations and meta-analysis of effect size differences. It's likely you will need to report moderator analyses in your results section (see Chap. 12).

I've reported moderator analyses using the format of your main analyses, focusing on overall effects for each category of your moderator or the overall effect if it is a continuous moderator. In Cooke et al. (2023), we found that sample type and time frame both moderated the overall effect of forming implementation intentions on weekly drinking. So, for sample type, which had two categories (university; community), we reported meta-analyses of the overall effect size for weekly drinking for each category separately. In other words, we computed a meta-analysis of effect size differences for the studies that recruited community samples and then separately, computed a meta-analysis of effect size differences for the studies that recruited university samples. We partitioned the effect sizes into these two categories. Results highlighted why we had a significant moderation effect: the effect size difference for community samples was $d_+ = -0.38$ (a small effect size difference), while the effect size difference for university samples was $d_+ = -0.04$ (a null effect size difference). Therefore, the same intervention—forming implementation intentions—had a significant effect on self-reported weekly drinking when received by community samples, and no effect on self-reported weekly drinking when received by university samples.

As well as reporting the overall effect sizes for each category, you should also report the homogeneity of the overall effect size and a test of difference between the categories, either a Z test of independent effects or a chi-square test (see Chap. 12 for more on tests). The reason for reporting the heterogeneity of the categorical effect sizes is to see if you have met one of the original goals of meta-analysis; to find a homogenous, overall effect size. Both effect sizes (those for community and university samples) lacked heterogeneity. This suggests that the significant effect of forming implementation intentions on weekly drinking in community samples is consistent. Conversely, the null effect size difference on weekly drinking for university students being homogenous suggests there's unlikely to be an effect of this intervention in university samples.

Narrative Synthesis

One of my favourite aspects of meta-analysis is that you need much less narrative synthesis than in a systematic review. The meta-analysis provides the data synthesis, meaning you can save your word count for other sections of the paper. I do not want to leave you with the impression that meta-analysis does away with narrative synthesis entirely, however. You still need to report key information.

For instance, if you were to only write the results of a meta-analysis as $r_+ = 0.45$ you are leaving a lot of useful information out. You've not told the reader what magnitude this result is (i.e. medium-sized correlation in Cohen (1992) terms). Similarly, if you report results as heterogeneous by writing $I^2 = 78\%$, what does that mean (i.e. high heterogeneity)? Or stating there is publication bias. Statistics can convey a lot of information on their own, but without being put into context by the author, they lose most of their value. After toiling for several months (years) on your meta-analysis you will have become an expert on the literature you are synthesising. This means you are well placed to explain to the reader, who is almost certainly less knowledgeable than you, what the results mean.

As I typically meta-analyse results from fields I know well, I have already invested considerable time in thinking about what the results would mean *before* I run the meta-analysis. When I started working on Cooke et al. (2016), I knew what I expected to find regarding theory of planned behaviour relationships for alcohol and was using the meta-analysis to test those expectations. Alternatively, when I began working on Cooke et al. (2023), I was curious to see how big the effect of implementation intentions on alcohol outcomes was. I suspected that results would show small effect size differences for drinking behaviour because, based on my reading of the alcohol literature, interventions to reduce drinking behaviour are typically associated with small effect size differences. As recommended in Chap. 7, it's advisable to get to know your included studies' effect sizes before running a meta-analysis to prime you for your meta-analysis output.

A Note on Figures, Tables, Supplementary Files, and the Open Science Framework

In most of my meta-analyses, I included a table (Cooke et al., 2023; Cooke & Sheeran, 2004) or tables (Cooke & French, 2008) containing information about the included studies in the main text. This is an invaluable source of information for you when writing up results of your meta-analysis as it contains all the key information you need when interpreting the results of your meta-analyses. These tables almost always include effect sizes and information that is important for moderator analyses, such as screening type (Cooke & French, 2008), or intervention type (Cooke et al., 2023).

Cooke et al. (2016) was the only paper that did not include such a table in the main text. The main reason this table was not included in the main text is that there were several other tables summarising results from main analyses and moderator analyses that I decided were more important to include. The table of studies was included as a Supplementary Table instead. Other tables I've included in the main body of the paper usually summarise results from moderator analyses. There tend to be a lot of statistics associated with these analyses, so, they are best displayed in a table.

Since Cooke et al. (2016), I've used PRISMA reporting (Liberati et al., 2009) guidelines in meta-analyses I've authored and included PRISMA flow diagrams as Fig. 1 in Cooke et al. (2016) and Cooke et al. (2023). You can include the PRISMA checklist as an appendix or supplementary table if you like, and I submit this document with the paper when I send it to a journal, but I don't think it's essential that the checklist is published in the main body of your text. In my opinion, the value of the checklist is to make sure YOU have included all the relevant information in your paper. Other figures to consider including in your main text are forest plots, meta-regression analyses, and funnel plots. Of these, I think that forest plots are the most useful to include in the main body of the paper. I tend to include visualisations of heterogeneity, from a meta-regression plot, or publication bias from a funnel plot, as supplementary files.

Rigorous reporting of meta-analyses can lead to lots of additional tables and figures, so include these as supplementary files. We had nine forest and nine funnel plots in Cooke et al. (2016), plus, three supplementary tables, one of which was the main table of information extracted from included studies. The other tables provided information on excluded studies and how we coded the patterns of consumption data for each study. Cooke et al.'s (2023) supplementary tables include how we coded the full factorial designs and a description of control conditions. We also included Figures generated in RevMan for risk of bias using the Cochrane Tool, so, tables displaying quality ratings can appear as supplementary tables.

The final thing to say in this section is that during the initial submission of Cooke et al. (2023), which was rejected by the journal we submitted the paper to, we had to upload the raw data used to calculate effect size differences to the Open Science Framework. This was stipulated by the journal we submitted to and strikes me as good practice AND allows you to save space in your paper. As noted repeatedly, authors of experiments/interventions in the psychological literature rarely report computed effect sizes, so for transparent reporting in a paper, you would have to report the raw mean and standard deviations for both groups, plus both sample sizes, in your table of included studies. That's six columns immediately!!! I recommend you put the raw statistics in a spreadsheet on the Open Science Framework, like we did, and report the computed effect size differences in the paper. Then you only need three columns—the effect size difference and sample sizes for each group.

Putting the extracted raw statistics on the Open Science Framework means anyone can check your calculations. This might seem scary, but, the alternative, of review teams calculating effect size differences then pooling them using meta-analysis does not sound much better to me—and I speak as someone who used to do this!!! It's better to fear someone finding an error in your working than someone NOT finding an error in your working. If someone finds the error it can be corrected, if undiscovered, it's unlikely it ever will be.

Discussion

Like papers reporting results from a primary analysis, the opening paragraph of the discussion in a meta-analysis paper should contain a summary of the main findings. The second paragraph contains text comparing results from the meta-analysis to the broader literature. In Cooke and French (2008), Cooke et al. (2016), and Cooke et al. (2023), I pretty much did the same thing—compare the results of the meta-analysis I was writing about with similar meta-analyses reported in the literature. While Cooke and French's text compares results from meta-analysis of screening relationships to broader meta-analyses of theory of planned behaviour/theory of reasoned action meta-analyses (e.g. Armitage & Conner, 2001), publication of more specific meta-analyses allowed me to make more focused comparisons in Cooke et al. (2016) and Cooke et al. (2023). In the former, I compared results for alcohol studies to McEachan's et al.'s (2011) meta-analysis of health behaviours and Topa and Moriano's (2010) meta-analysis of theory of planned behaviour smoking studies. In the latter, I compared the effect size difference we found for alcohol with equivalent pooled effect size differences for physical activity (Bélanger-Gravel et al., 2013) and dietary behaviours (Vilà et al., 2017). Comparing meta-analytic results with other meta-analytic results allows for a neat comparison; however, you may be meta-analysing a literature where other meta-analyses do not exist for such a comparison or where metas exist but have used different methods/measures to those you have pooled. In this case, I recommend directly comparing your meta-analytic findings to results from existing papers on the same topic. Although not ideal, as your meta-analysis is based on pooled data, such a comparison will still allow you to take the temperature of the research literature and draw out broader conclusions.

If you have more than one outcome, it's likely you'll need to discuss results for these in separate paragraphs, though this might depend on how similar the results are for the outcomes. In Cooke et al. (2023), the third and fourth paragraphs discussed why the meta-analysis of heavy episodic drinking studies yielded a null overall effect size difference.

Having compared the overall effect sizes relative to the broader literature, my discussions sections next discussed what moderator results mean. After discussing moderator effects in Cooke et al. (2016), we went on to discuss the novel finding that how perceived behavioural control was operationalised appears to affect the size of the correlation with intentions and behaviour. This was not a moderator analysis, but the idea was like testing a moderator effect, so we put this discussion at this point.

The remainder of the discussion follows the usual format for an academic paper in psychology. We have limitations or strengths and weaknesses, gaps in the literature, implications, sub-sections. One thing that is worth noting is that in the strengths and weaknesses section, I think it is reasonable to include both strengths and weaknesses of the included studies as well as strengths and weaknesses of the meta-analysis. A common weakness of meta-analysis is a lack of studies reporting tests of the same effect size, which limits moderator analyses. Other weaknesses can relate to the quality of included studies, or the reliability or validity of the measures used. I think it's valuable to highlight these weaknesses, plus strengths, across a literature as it helps researchers design and develop better tests of effect sizes in future studies. I always end my papers with a conclusion that sets out the takeaway messages for the reader. This is true of all my meta-analyses too.

Summary

The aim of this chapter was to offer guidance on how to write up the results of a meta-analysis for submission to a peer-review publication. I focused on how to write up results for a secondary analysis, drawing attention to key differences in reporting methods and results.

References

Armitage, C. J., & Conner, M. (2001). Efficacy of the theory of planned behaviour: A meta-analytic review. *British Journal of Social Psychology, 40*(4), 471–499. https://doi.org/10.1348/014466601164939

Bélanger-Gravel, A., Godin, G., & Amireault, S. (2013). A meta-analytic review of the effect of implementation intentions on physical activity. *Health Psychology Review, 7*, 23–54. https://doi.org/10.1080/17437199.2011.560095

Borenstein, M., Hedges, L. V., Higgins, J. P. T., & Rothstein, H. R. (2005). *Comprehensive Meta-Analysis* (Version 2) [Computer software]. Biostat.

Cohen, J. (1992). A power primer. *Psychological Bulletin, 112*(1), 155–159.

Conner, M., Warren, R., Close, S., & Sparks, P. (1999). Alcohol consumption and the theory of planned behavior: An examination of the cognitive mediation of past behaviorid. *Journal of Applied Social Psychology, 29*(8), 1676–1704. https://doi.org/10.1111/j.1559-1816.1999.tb02046.x

Cooke, R., Dahdah, M., Norman, P., & French, D. P. (2016). How well does the theory of planned behaviour predict alcohol consumption? A systematic review and meta-analysis. *Health Psychology Review, 10*, 148–167. https://doi.org/10.1080/17437199.2014.947547

Cooke, R., & French, D. P. (2008). How well do the theory of reasoned action and theory of planned behaviour predict intentions and attendance at screening programmes? A meta-analysis. *Psychology & Health, 23*(7), 745–765. https://doi.org/10.1080/08870440701544437

Cooke, R., & French, D. P. (2011). The role of context and timeframe in moderating relationships within the theory of planned behaviour. *Psychology & Health, 26*(9), 1225–1240. https://doi.org/10.1080/08870446.2011.572260

Cooke, R., McEwan, H., & Norman, P. (2023). The effect of forming implementation intentions on alcohol consumption: A systematic review and meta-analysis. *Drug and Alcohol Review, 42*, 68–80. https://doi.org/10.1111/dar.13553

Cooke, R., & Sheeran, P. (2004). Moderation of cognition-intention and cognition-behaviour relations: A meta-analysis of properties of variables from the theory of planned behaviour. *The British Journal of Social Psychology, 43*(Pt 2), 159–186. https://doi.org/10.1348/0144666041501688

Hunter, J. E., Schmidt, F., & Jackson, G. B. (1982). *Meta-analysis: Cumulating research findings across studies*. SAGE.

Liberati, A., Altman, D. G., Tetzlaff, J., Mulrow, C., Gøtzsche, P. C., Ioannidis, J. P. A., Clarke, M., Devereaux, P. J., Kleijnen, J., & Moher, D. (2009). The PRISMA statement for reporting systematic reviews and meta-analyses of studies that evaluate health care interventions: Explanation and elaboration. *Journal of Clinical Epidemiology, 62*, e1–e34. https://doi.org/10.1016/j.jclinepi.2009.06.006

Malaguti, A., Ciocanel, O., Sani, F., Dillon, J. F., Eriksen, A., & Power, K. (2020). Effectiveness of the use of implementation intentions on reduction of substance use: A meta-analysis. *Drug and Alcohol Dependence, 214*, 108120. https://doi.org/10.1016/j.drugalcdep.2020.108120

McEachan, R. R. C., Conner, M., Taylor, N. J., & Lawton, R. J. (2011). Prospective prediction of health-related behaviours with the theory of planned behaviour: A meta-analysis. *Health Psychology Review, 5*, 97–144. https://doi.org/10.1080/17437199.2010.521684

Morris, S. B. (2008). Estimating effect sizes from pretest-posttest-control group designs. *Organizational Research Methods, 11*(2), 364–386. https://doi.org/10.1177/1094428106291059

Norman, P., Cameron, D., Epton, T., Webb, T. L., Harris, P. R., Millings, A., & Sheeran, P. (2018). A randomized controlled trial of a brief online intervention to reduce alcohol consumption in new university students: Combining self-affirmation, theory of planned behaviour messages, and implementation intentions. *British Journal of Health Psychology, 23*(1), 108–127. https://doi.org/10.1111/bjhp.12277

Rosenthal, R. R. (1979). The File drawer problem and tolerance for null results. *Psychological Bulletin, 86*, 638–641.

Schwarzer, R. (1988). *Meta: Programs for secondary data analysis.* [Computer Software].

Sheeran, P., & Orbell, S. (1998). Do intentions predict condom use? Meta-analysis and examination of six moderator variables. *British Journal of Social Psychology, 37*(2), 231–250. https://doi.org/10.1111/j.2044-8309.1998.tb01167.x

Topa, G., & Moriano, L. J. A. (2010). Theory of planned behavior and smoking: Meta-analysis and SEM model. *Substance Abuse and Rehabiliation, 1*, 23–33.

Vilà, I., Carrero, I., & Redondo, R. (2017). Reducing fat intake using implementation intentions: A meta-analytic review. *British Journal of Health Psychology, 22*, 281–294. https://doi.org/10.1111/bjhp.12230

Glossary

Bounded A statistic that must fall within a certain range of values.

Confidence intervals Statistics that represent a range of possible values an effect size can take. Typically covers 95% of all possible values the effect size could take.

Correlation Summary statistic that tests the linear association between two variables.

Cross-sectional Study design where data is collected on one occasion.

d_+ Notation used to denote the sample-weighted average effect size difference.

Dispersion How values on a variable are spread across a dataset. Variance and standard deviation are statistics used to assess dispersion.

Effect size Summary statistic that represents results from a sample. Correlations and effect size differences are types of effect sizes.

Effect size difference A summary statistic that represents the difference in mean scores on an outcome between two groups having accounted for dispersion in scores for each group.

Fixed-effect meta-analysis A type of meta-analysis that assumes all included studies have the same 'true' effect size and only vary in the precision with which it is measured.

Forest plot Graph used to visualise effect sizes included in a meta-analysis. Individual effect sizes are represented by squares, with lines showing confidence intervals either side of the square. A diamond at the bottom of the plot represents the overall effect size.

Funnel plot Graph used to visualise dispersion of effect sizes around the overall effect size. Used to show asymmetry in the reporting of effect sizes to identify publication bias.

Grey literature Sources, such as datasets, reports, and theses, not published in peer-review journals.

Heterogeneity When effect sizes in a set of included studies significantly differ from one another. The opposite of homogeneity.

R. Cooke, *Meta-Analysis for Psychologists*,
https://doi.org/10.1007/978-3-031-73773-2

Homogeneity When effect sizes in a set of included studies do not significantly differ from one another. The opposite of heterogeneity.

Independent groups design A design where at least two groups of participants are recruited and are treated differently in one or more ways.

I^2 A measure of heterogeneity between effect sizes.

Longitudinal design Study design where data is collected on multiple occasions, often several months apart.

MAJOR Jamovi plugin that runs the metafor software package.

Mean difference Difference between two groups' means on the same variable.

metafor A software package for running meta-analysis in R.

Moderator A variable tested in a moderator analysis in an attempt to reduce heterogeneity in results.

Moderator (sub-group) analysis Analysis testing the idea that effect sizes vary as a function of a moderator variable.

Multicollinearity (collinearity) Principle that when variables are highly correlated (usually $r >= 0.80$) they are not independent of one another and unlikely to add unique variance to a regression model that includes both.

Negative correlation Correlation where as scores on one variable increase, scores on the other decrease. Sometimes called an inverse relationship.

Negative effect size difference An effect size difference that shows the control group scores better on the outcome relative to the intervention (or experimental) group.

Null correlation A correlation that shows there is no linear association between the variables.

Null effect size difference An effect size difference that shows no difference on the outcome between the intervention (experimental) and control groups.

Open Science Framework A website dedicated to increased replicability of results and transparency of reporting.

Overall effect size Summary statistic output by a meta-analysis. Represents the effect sizes for included studies after sample-weighting and averaging.

p-hacking Practice of repeatedly running significance tests with the goal of identifying a significant effect.

Point estimate Synonym for overall effect size.

Pooling Aggregating results across multiple samples (see also synthesising)

Positive correlation A correlation where as scores on one variables increase, so do scores on the other variable.

Positive effect size difference An effect size difference that shows the intervention (or experimental) group scores better on the outcome relative to the control group.

Primary study A study where the authors collected data themselves.

PRISMA Reporting standard for systematic reviews and meta-analyses.

Prospective design Type of longitudinal study design where data is collected on at least two occasions, often within several weeks.

PROSPERO An online register of systematic reviews.

Publication bias Tendency for academic journals to favour publication of studies reporting significant results.

Q (statistic) A measure of heterogeneity that compares the observed variation in effect sizes to the expected variation in effect sizes.

r_+ Notation used to denote the sample-weighted average correlation.

Randomised controlled trials (RCTs) Study designed to answer an important clinical question conducted using high-quality study designs to reduce the risk that various biases affect interpretation of results.

Random-effects meta-analysis A type of meta-analysis that assumes included studies vary in their 'true' effect size, meaning that each study should be weighted according to both the precision with which it is measured and variation in true effect sizes.

Sample error The difference between an effect size and the population mean.

Sample-weighting The process of assigning different weightings to studies included in a meta-analysis based on sample size: studies with larger samples are assigned greater weight relative to studies with smaller samples because studies with larger samples provide a more precise estimate of effect size.

Sample-weighted average correlation Overall effect size generated by a meta-analysis of correlations. Reported in text using r_+.

Sample-weighted average effect size difference Overall effect size generated by a meta-analysis of effect size differences. Reported in text using d_+.

Secondary study A study that reports a synthesis of results from multiple papers (samples) on the same topic. Meta-analyses and systematic reviews are both examples of secondary studies.

Sensitivity analysis A series of meta-analyses run to test the idea that the overall effect size is sensitive to the exclusion of any individual effect size.

Standardised mean difference Effect size that involves computing the difference in means between two groups while controlling for dispersion in means by pooling standard deviations. Synonymous with effect size difference and Cohen's (d).

Synthesising When you aggregate results across multiple samples (see also pooling).

Tau A statistic representing the standard deviation in true effect sizes.

Tau^2 A statistic representing the variance in true effect sizes.

Unbounded A statistic, like an effect size difference, that can take on any value.

Index

R. Cooke, *Meta-Analysis for Psychologists*,
https://doi.org/10.1007/978-3-031-73773-2

The manufacturer's authorised representative in the EU is Springer Nature Customer Service Centre GmbH, Europaplatz 3, 69115 Heidelberg, Germany. If you have any concerns regarding our products, please contact ProductSafety@springernature.com

Printed and bound by CPI Group (UK) Ltd, Croydon, CR0 4YY
09/06/2026
02132388-0001